AF251873

A NEW KIND OF BEAUTY

A NEW KIND OF BEAUTY

Phillip Toledano

with an essay by
W.M. Hunt

DEWI LEWIS PUBLISHING

I BELIEVE WE ARE AT THE VANGUARD OF A PERIOD OF HUMAN-INDUCED EVOLUTION. A TURNING POINT IN HISTORY WHERE WE ARE BEGINNING TO DEFINE NOT ONLY OUR OWN CONCEPT OF BEAUTY, BUT OF PHYSICALITY ITSELF. BEAUTY HAS ALWAYS BEEN A CURRENCY, AND NOW THAT WE FINALLY HAVE THE TECHNOLOGICAL MEANS TO MINT OUR OWN, WHAT CHOICES DO WE MAKE? IS BEAUTY INFORMED BY CONTEMPORARY CULTURE? BY HISTORY? OR IS IT DEFINED BY THE SURGEON'S HAND? WHEN WE RE-MAKE OURSELVES, ARE WE REVEALING OUR TRUE CHARACTER, OR ARE WE STRIPPING AWAY OUR VERY IDENTITY?

PHILLIP TOLEDANO

Steve

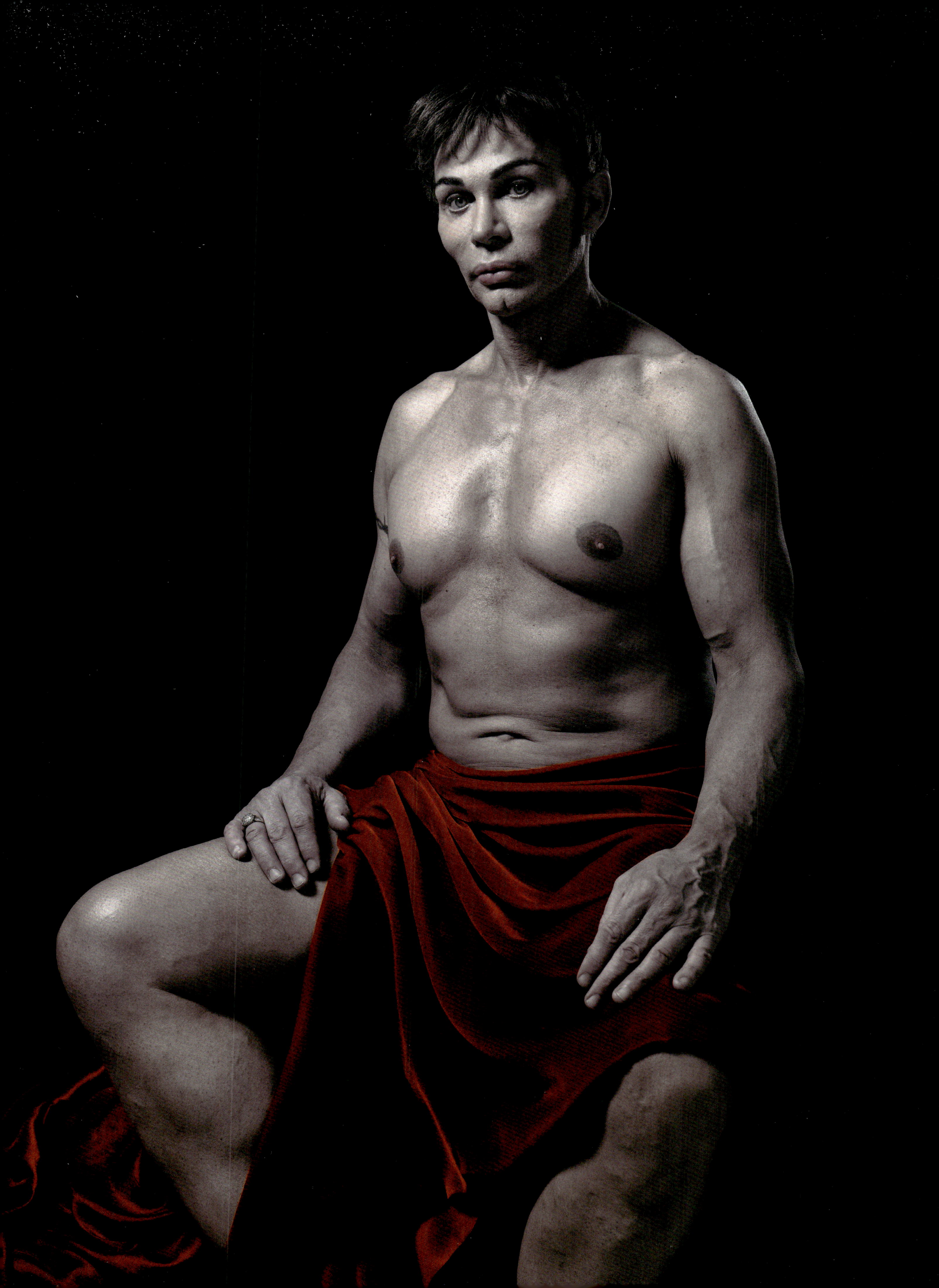

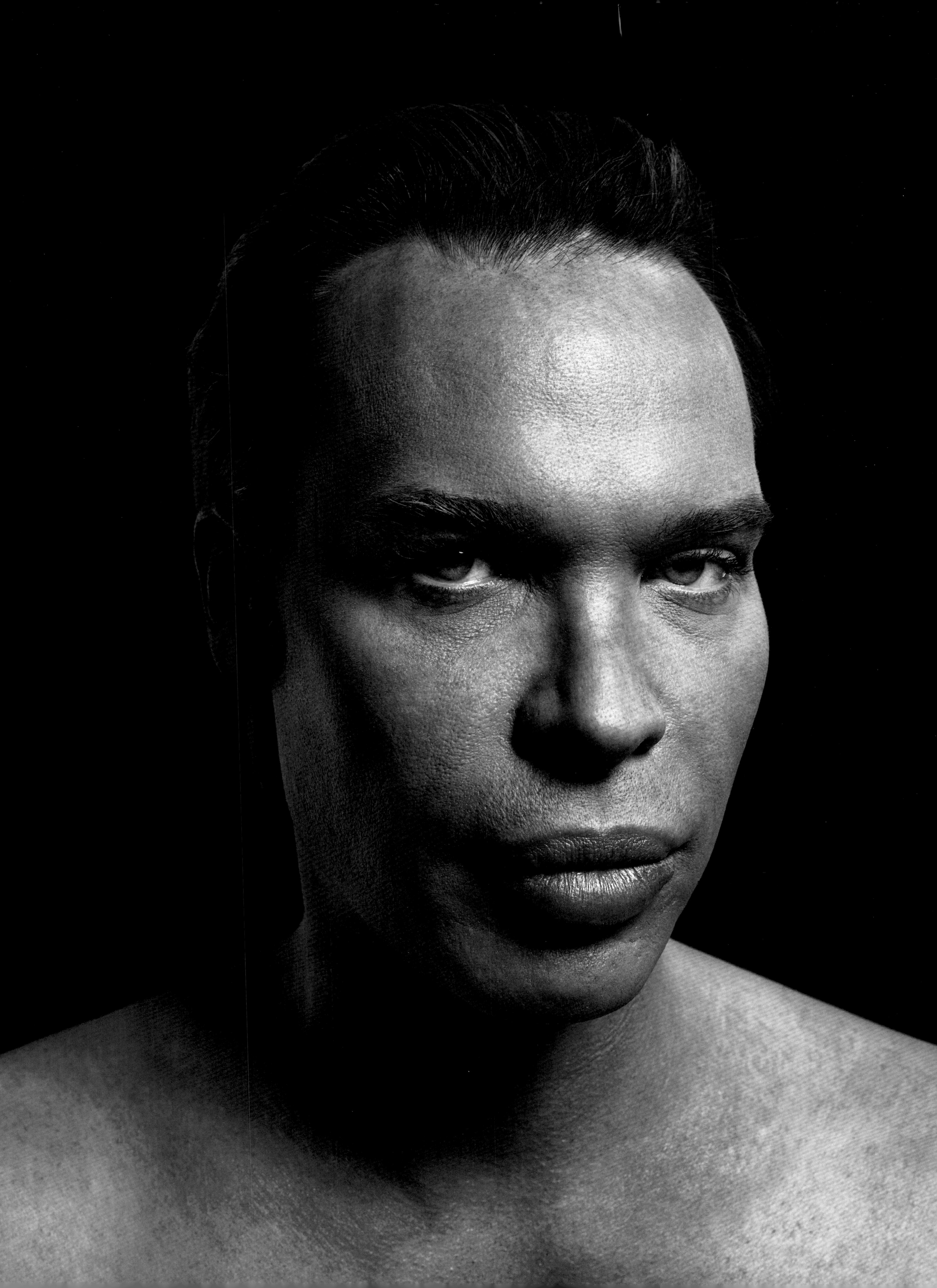

Ashley

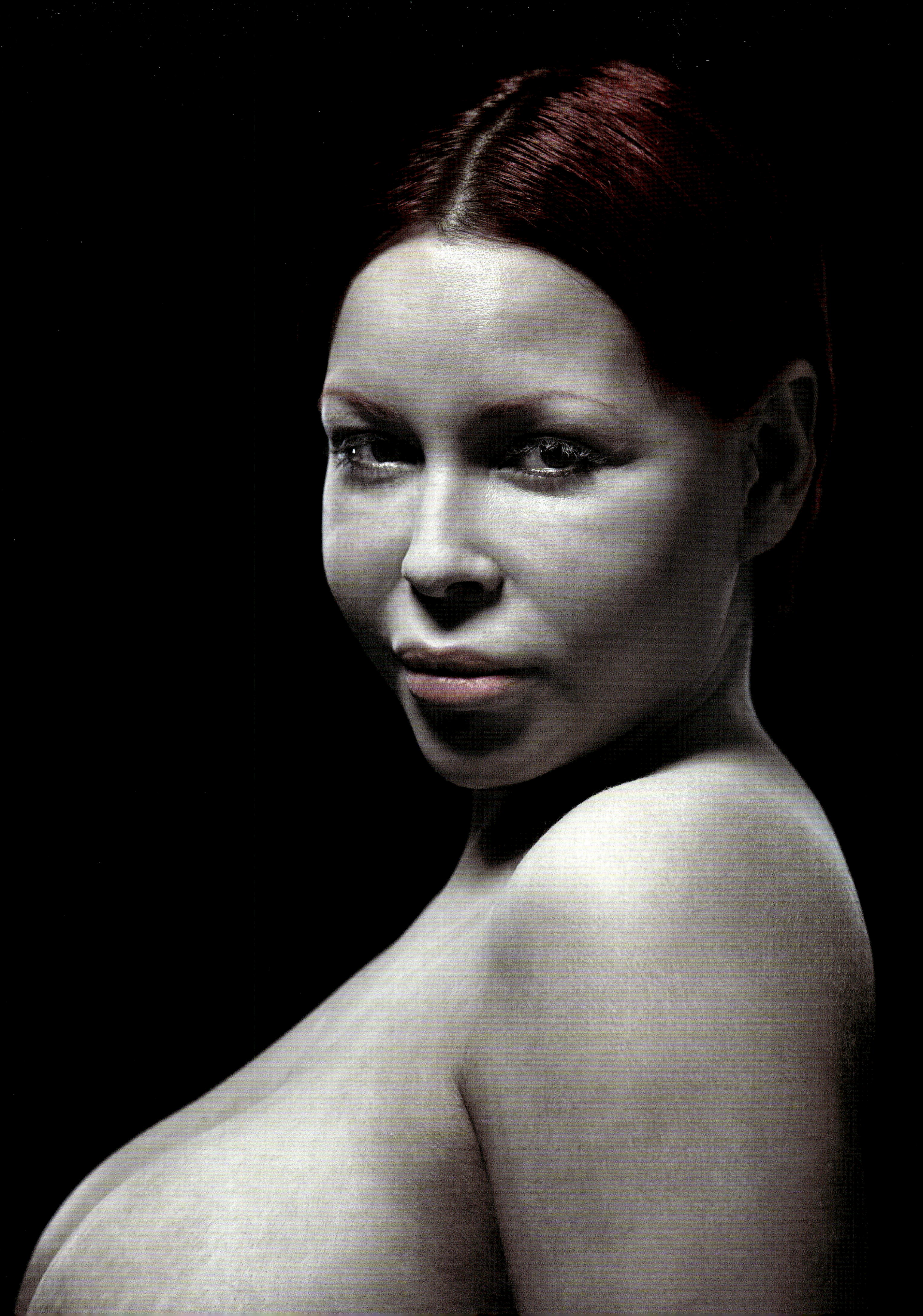

Justin

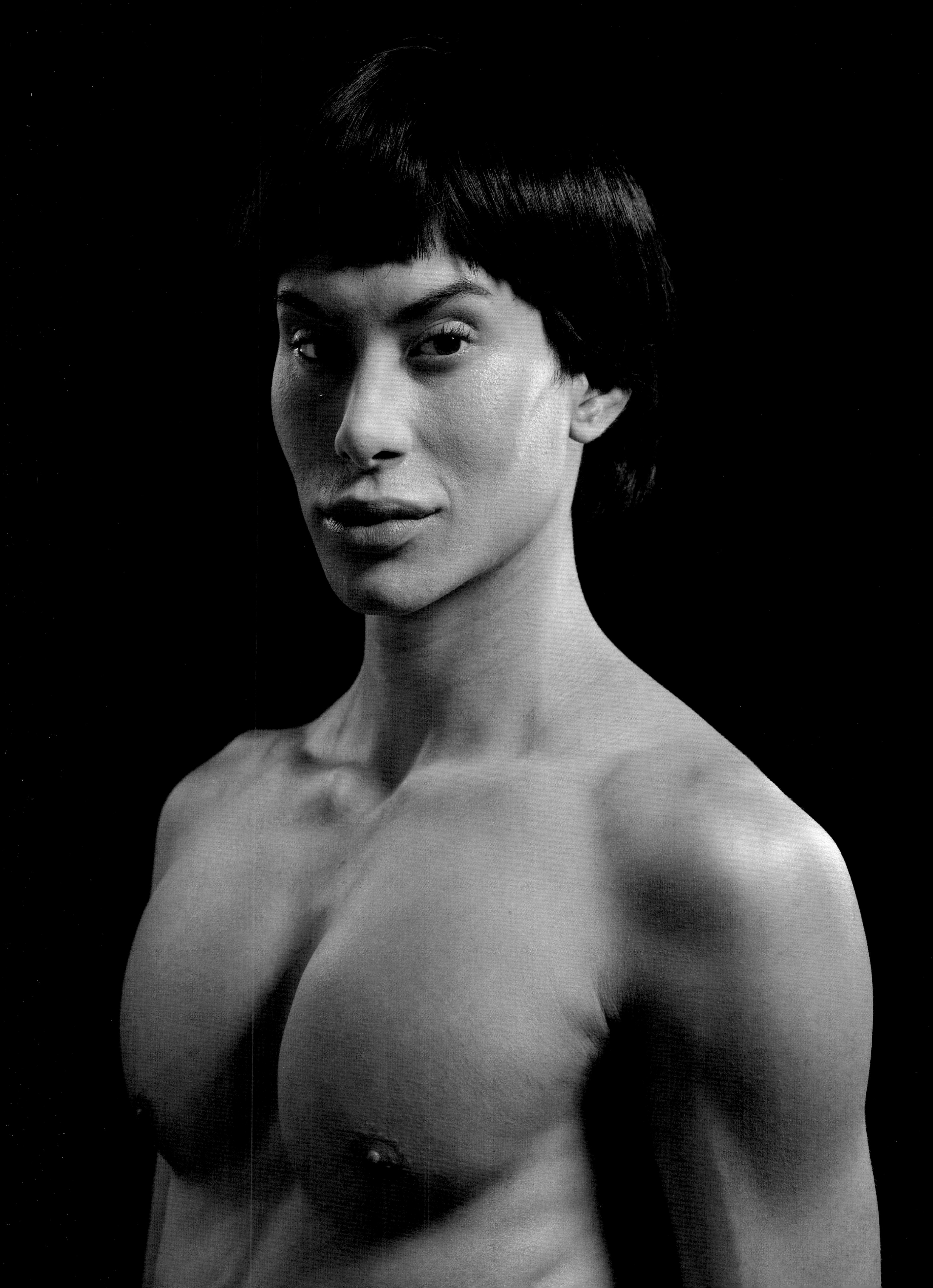

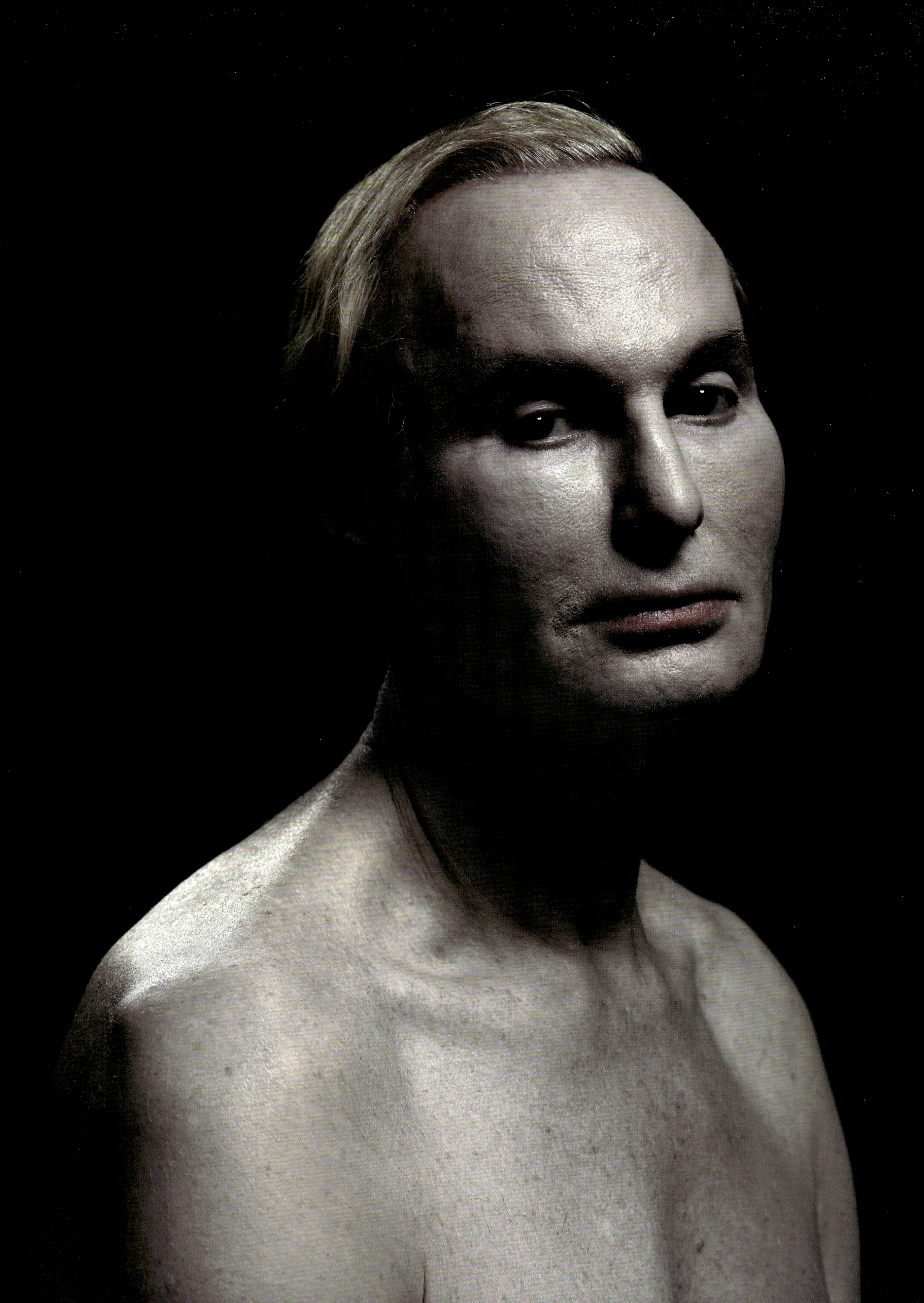

Fred

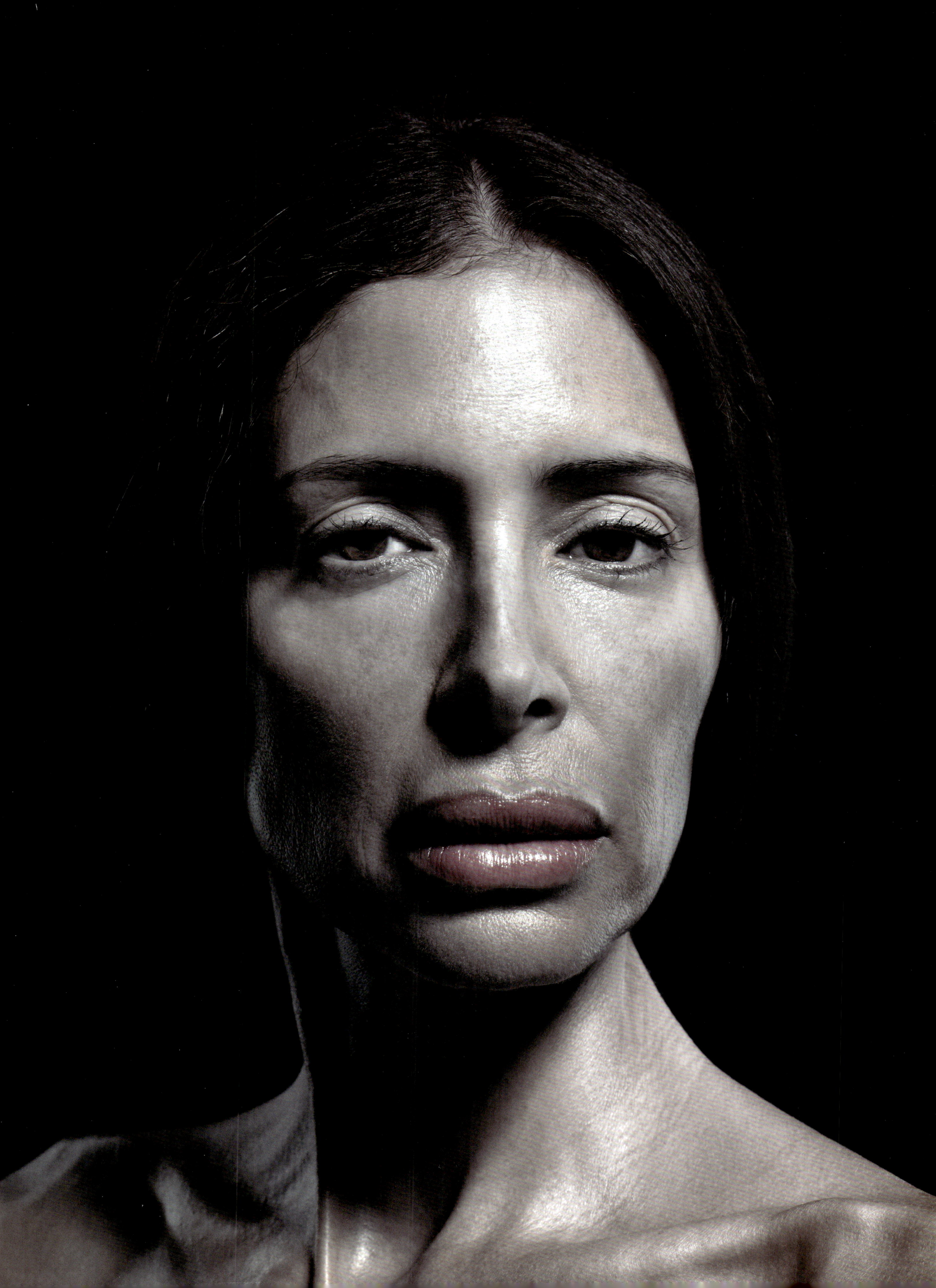

Ava

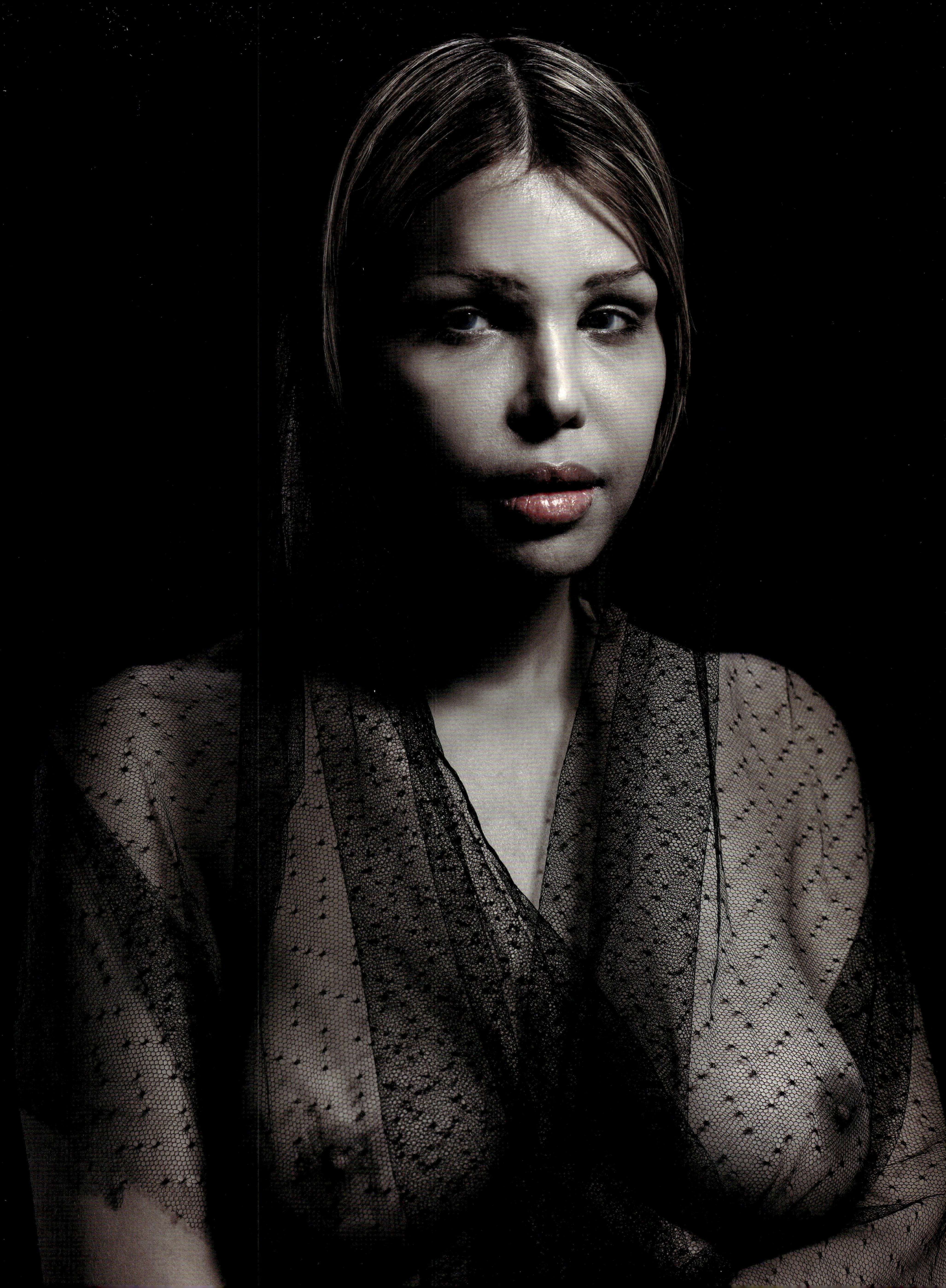

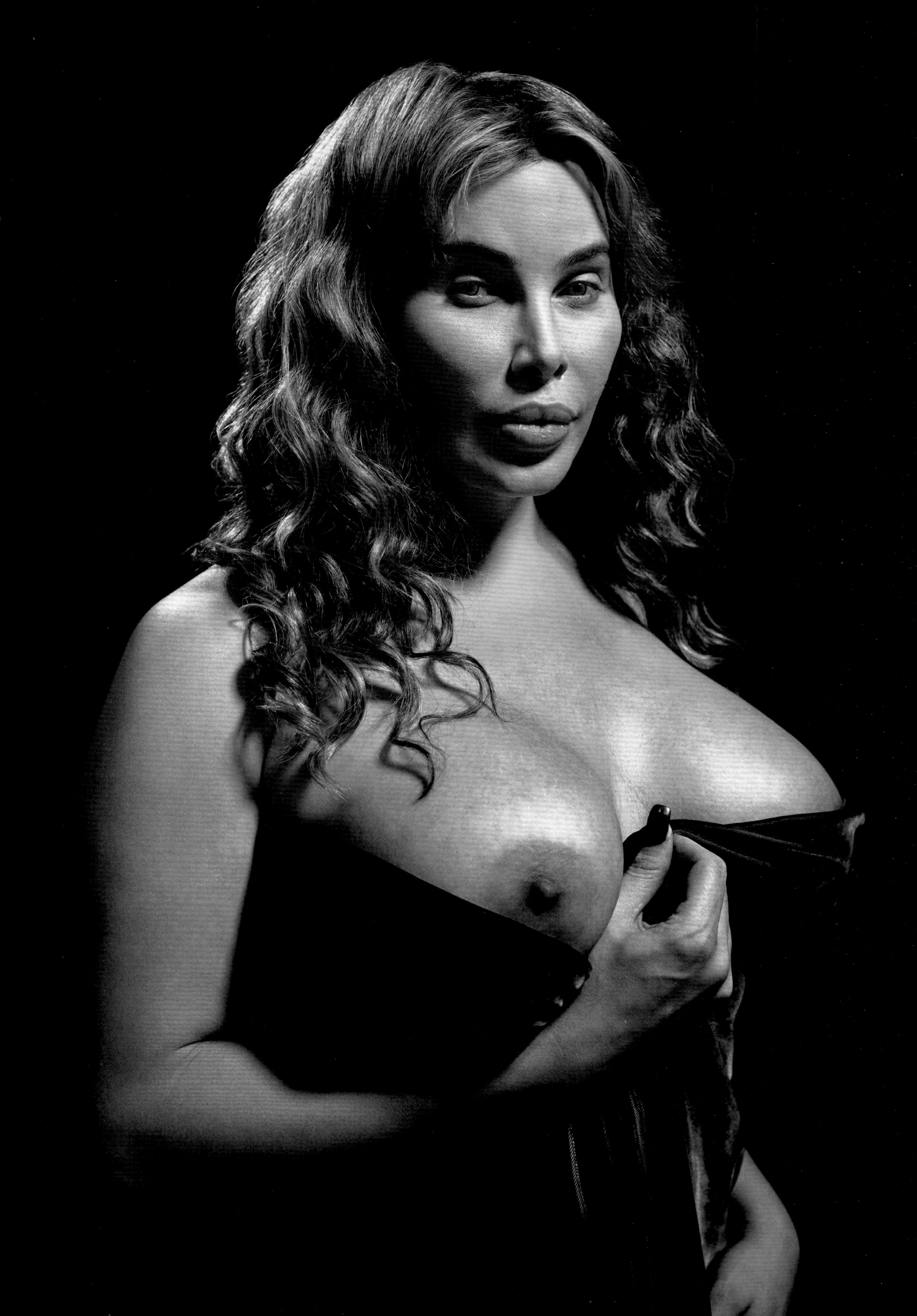

Dina – *following page* Monique

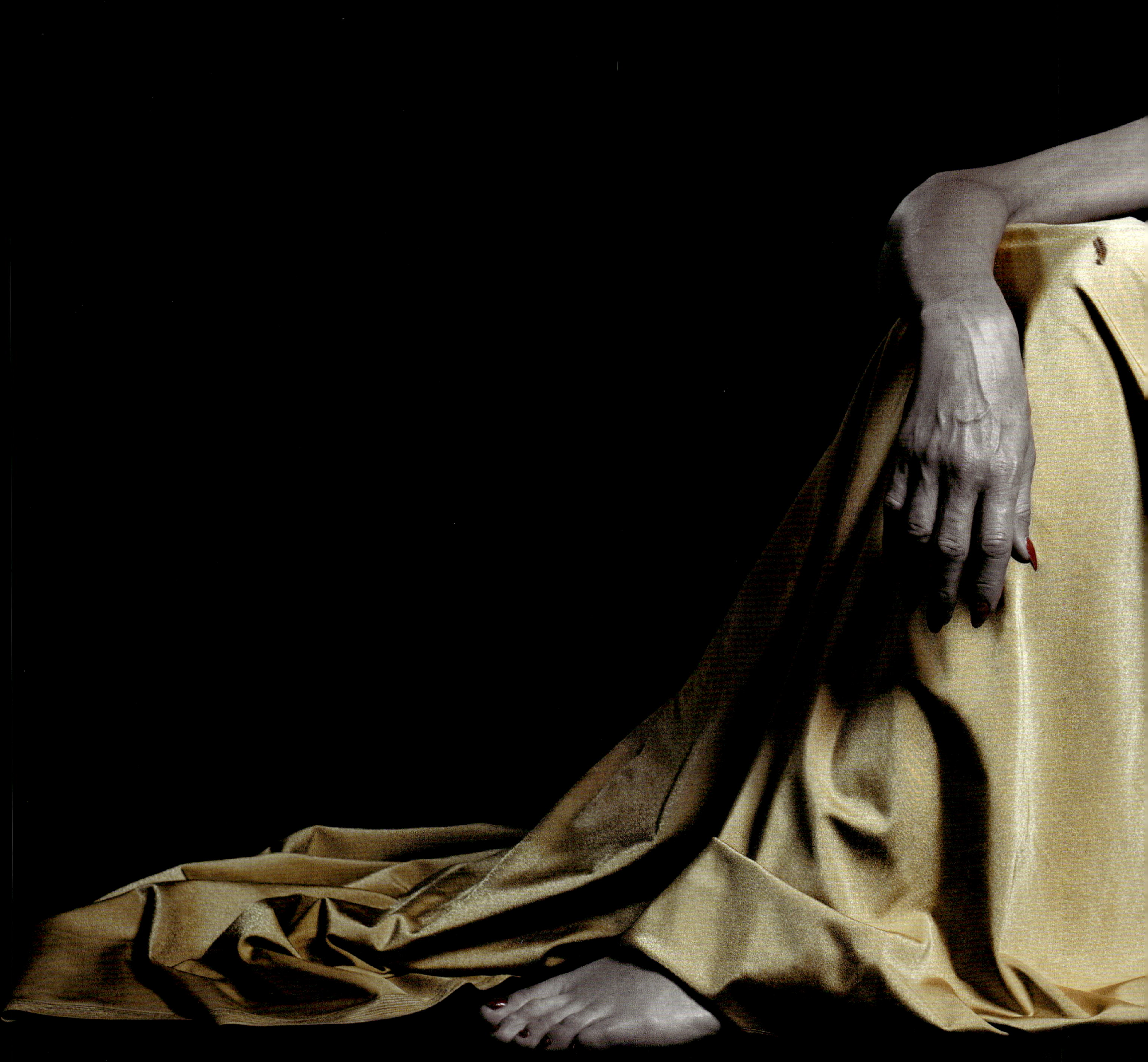

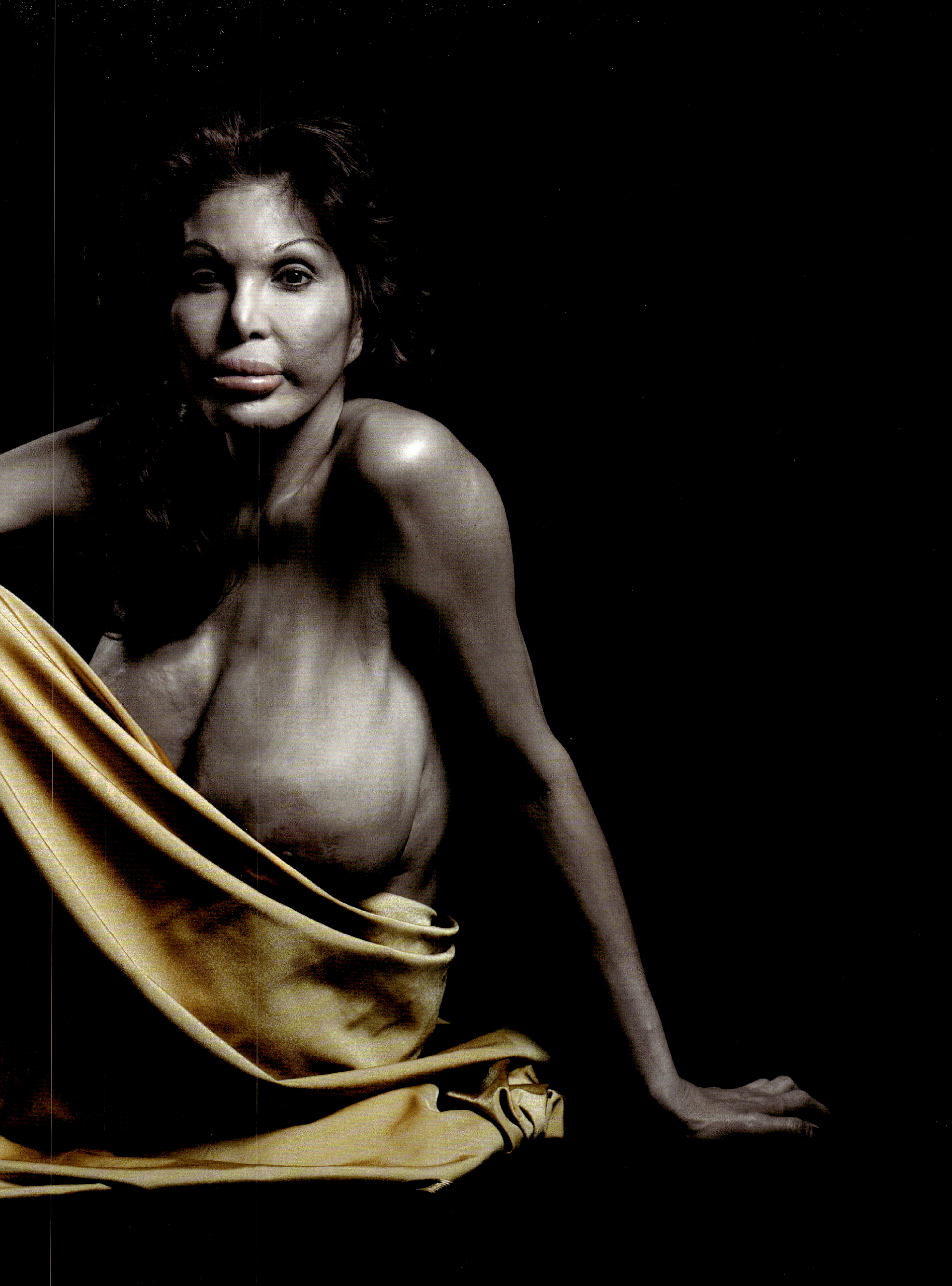

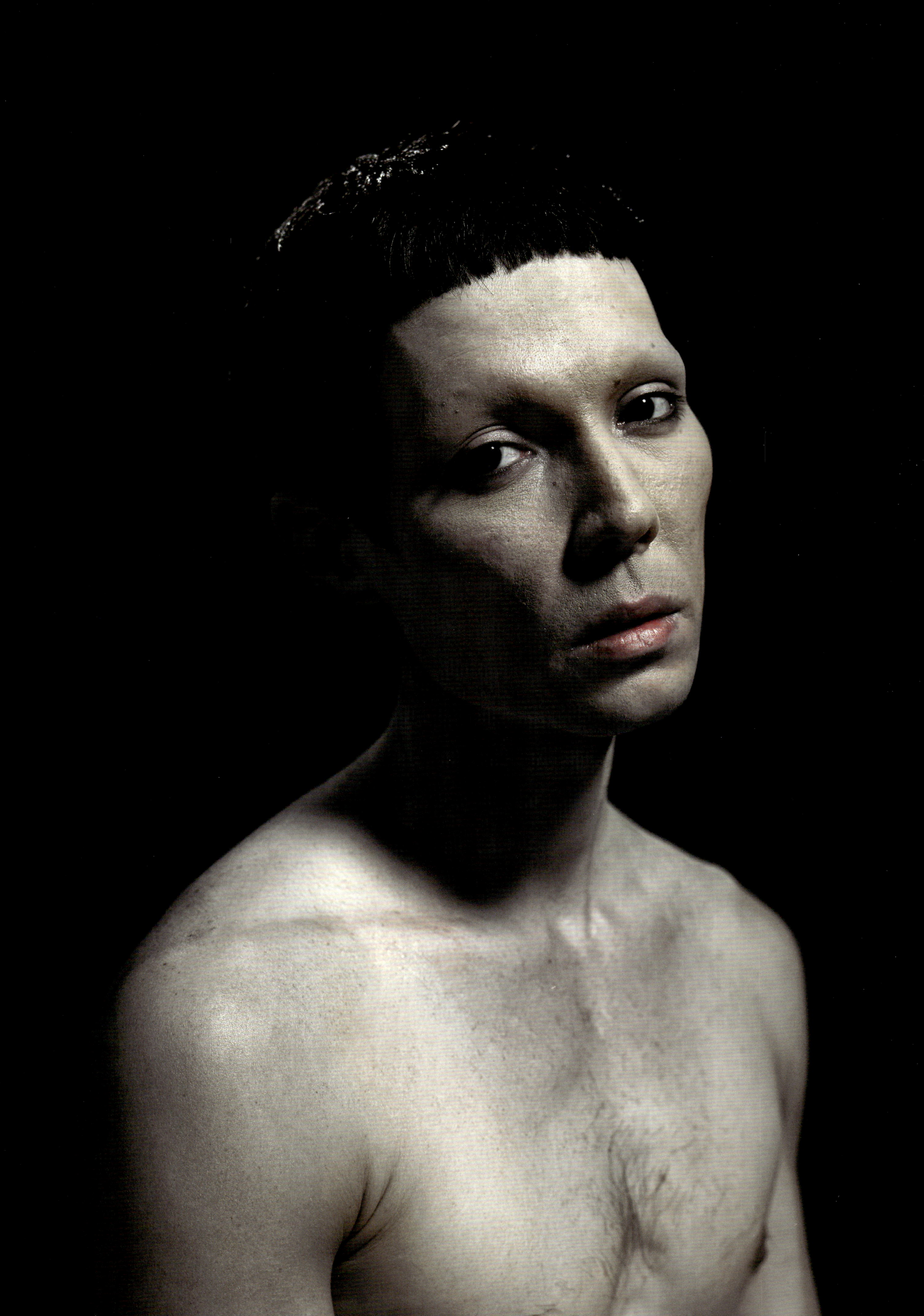

Michael

Jason

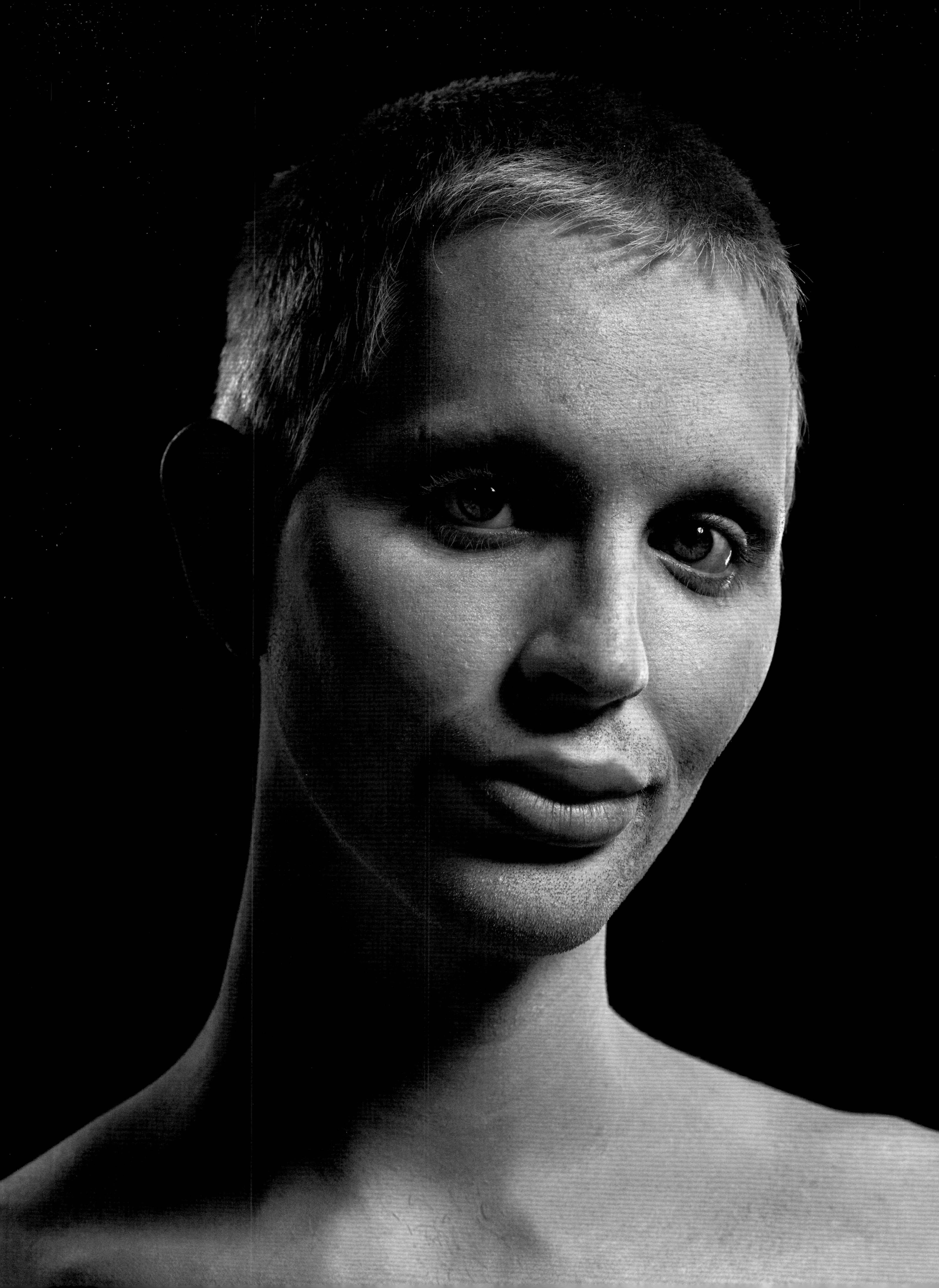

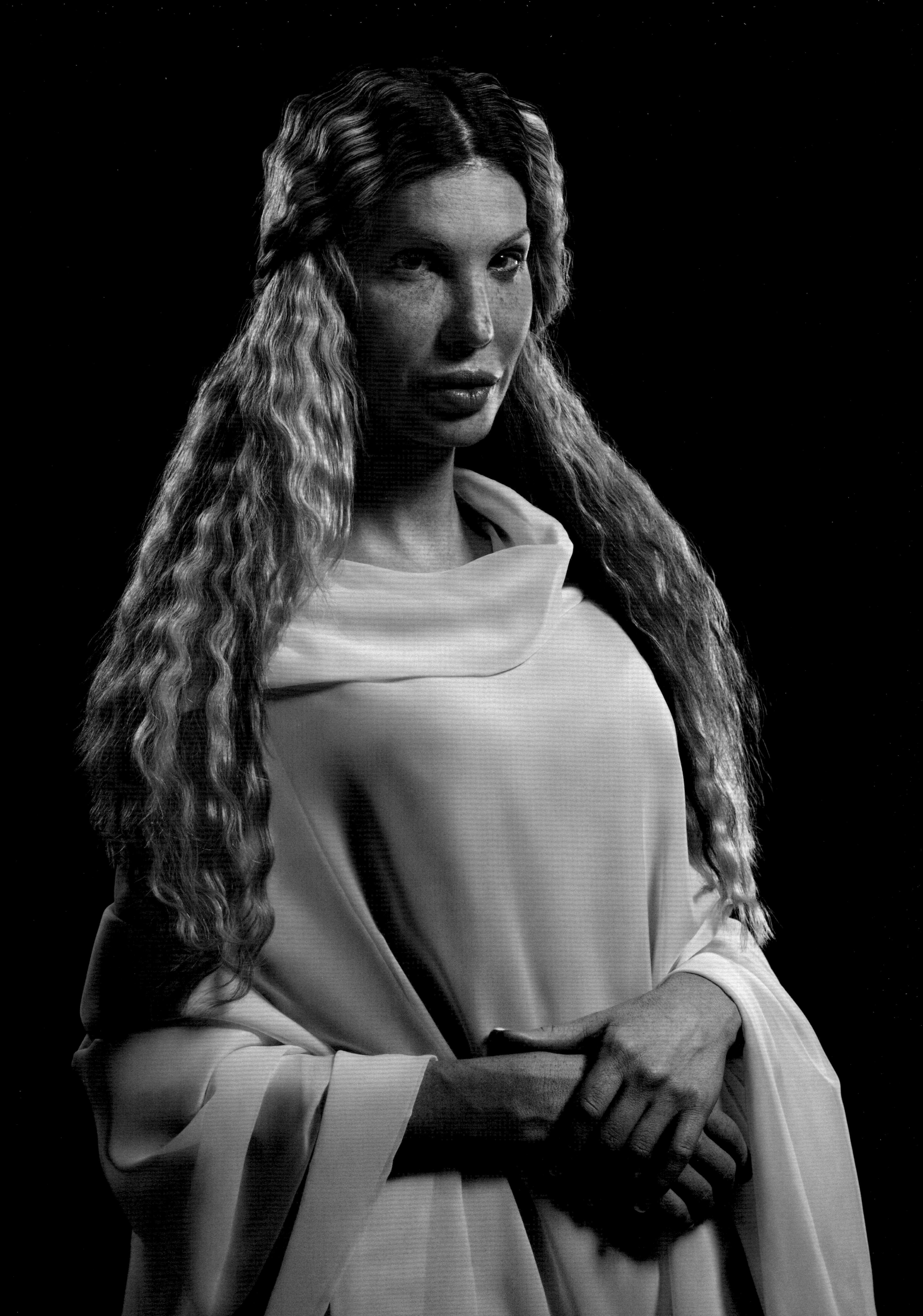

Nikki

Louis

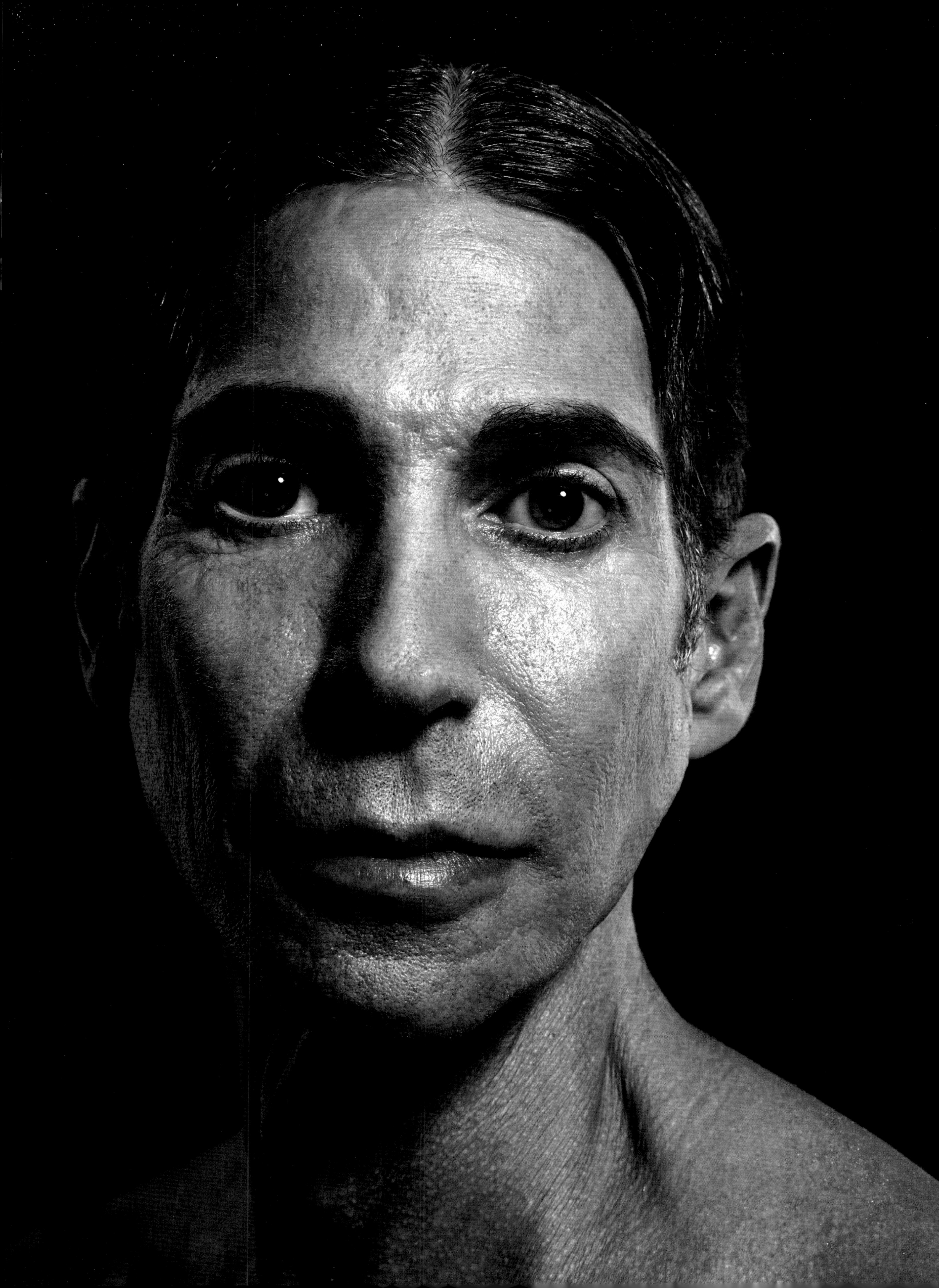

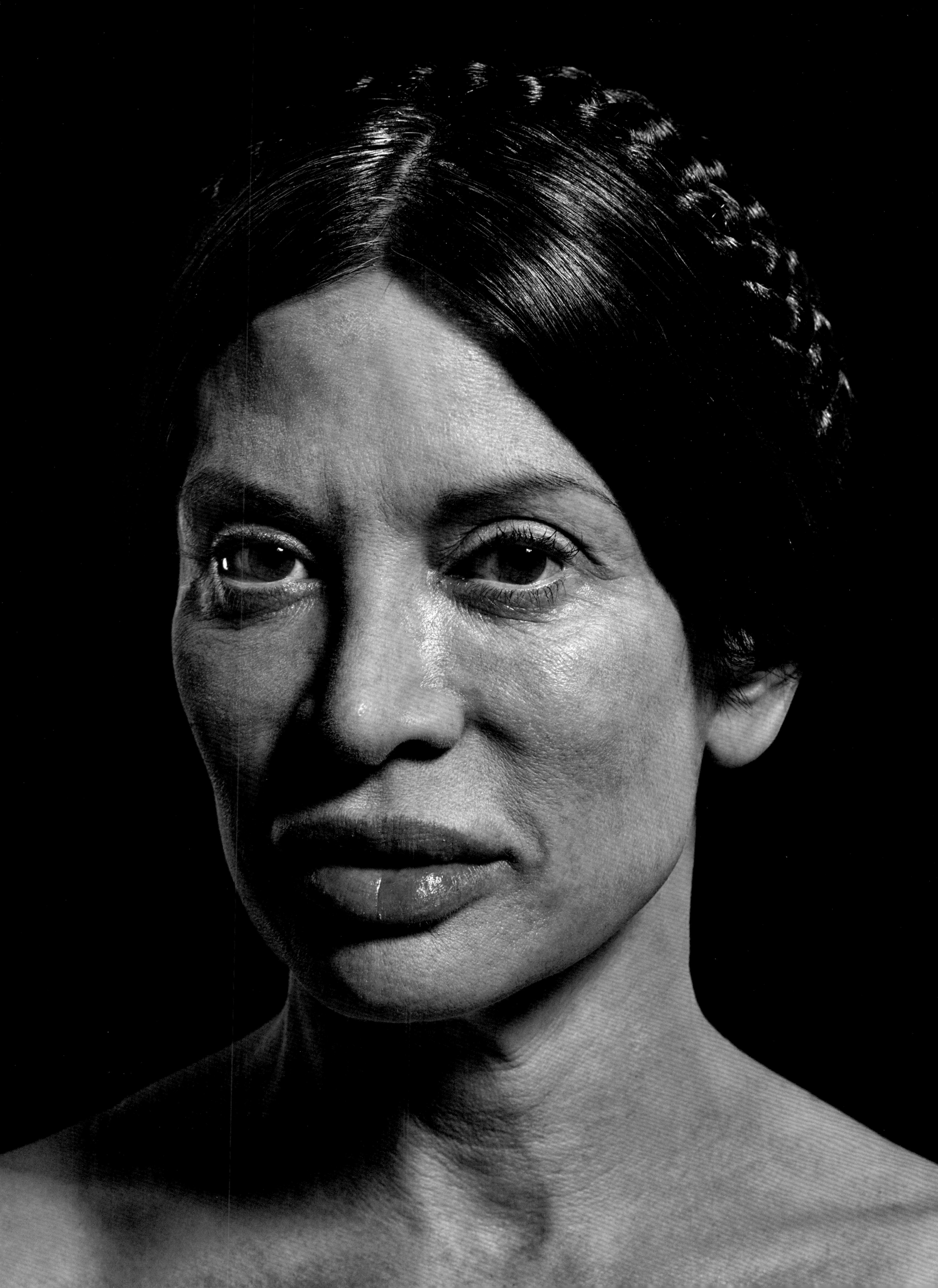

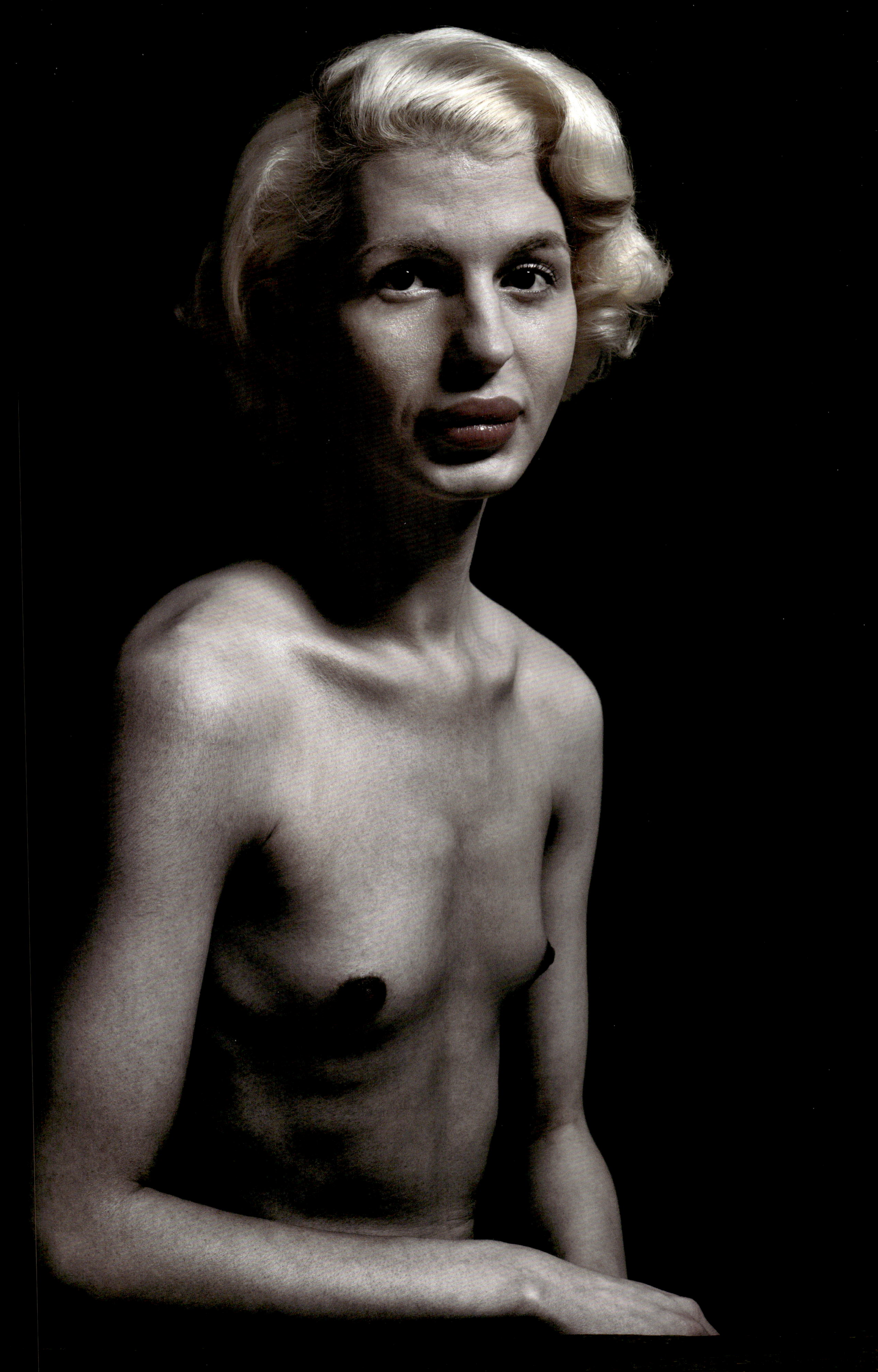

Paris

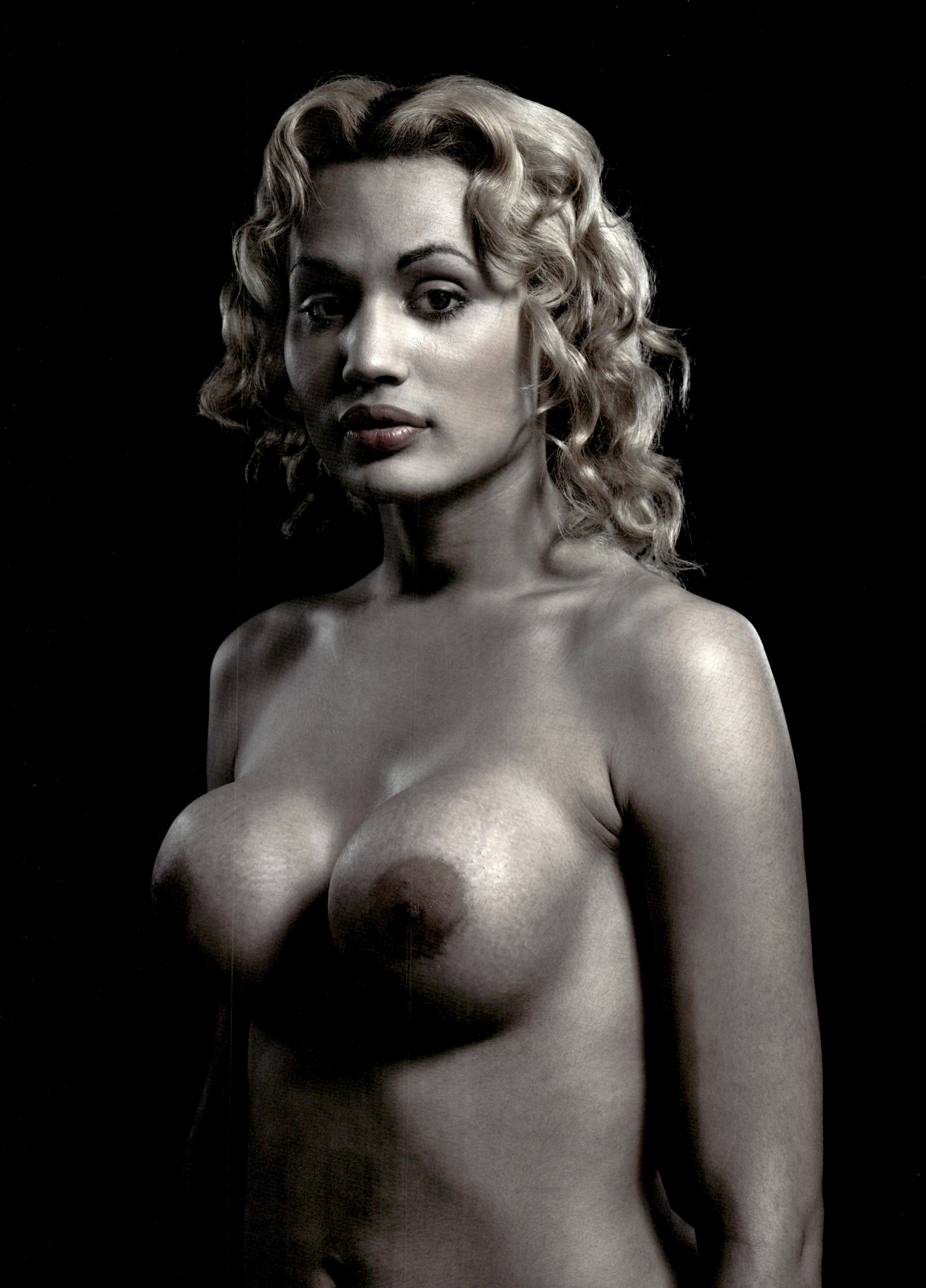

Sharon

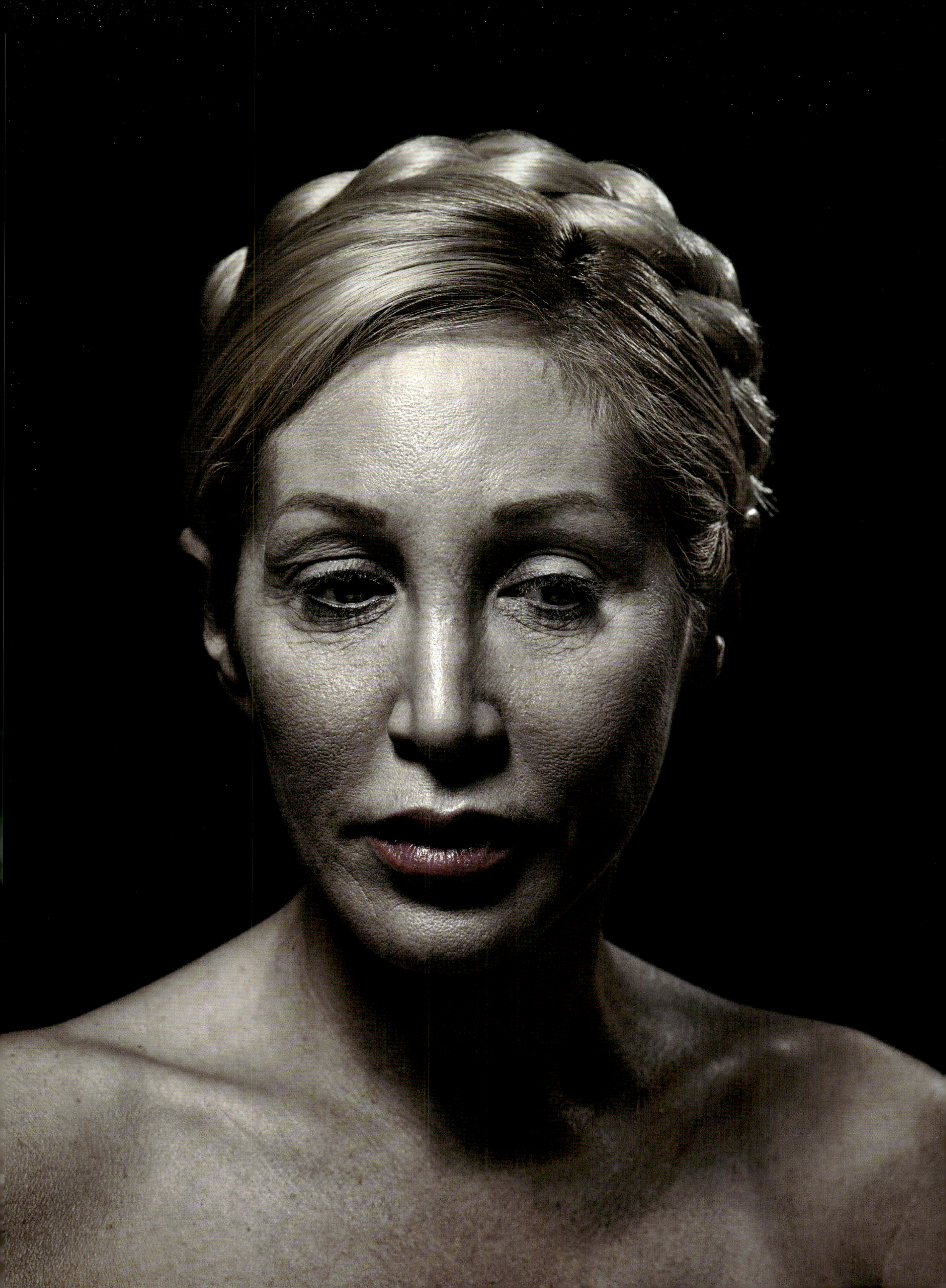

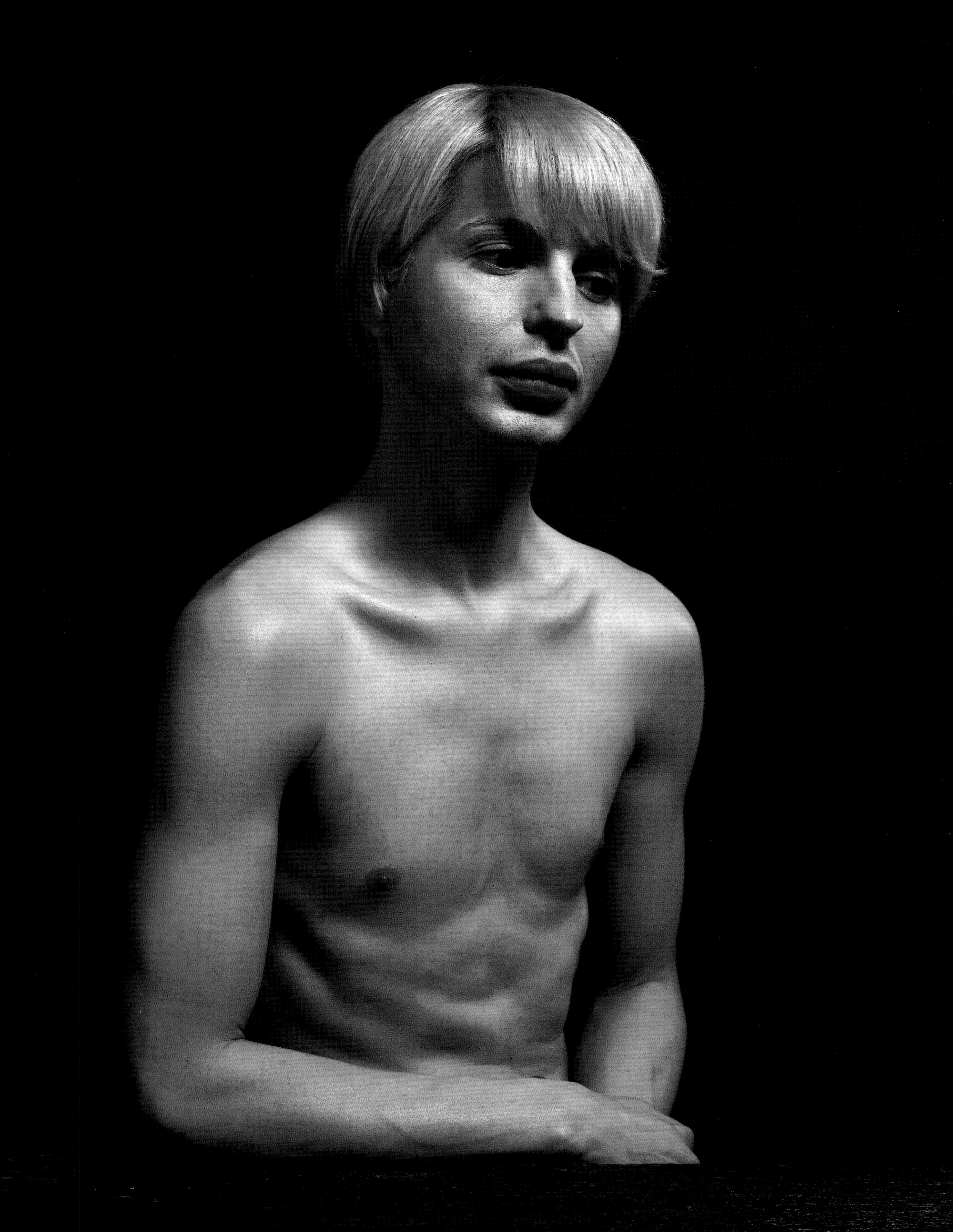

Kenny

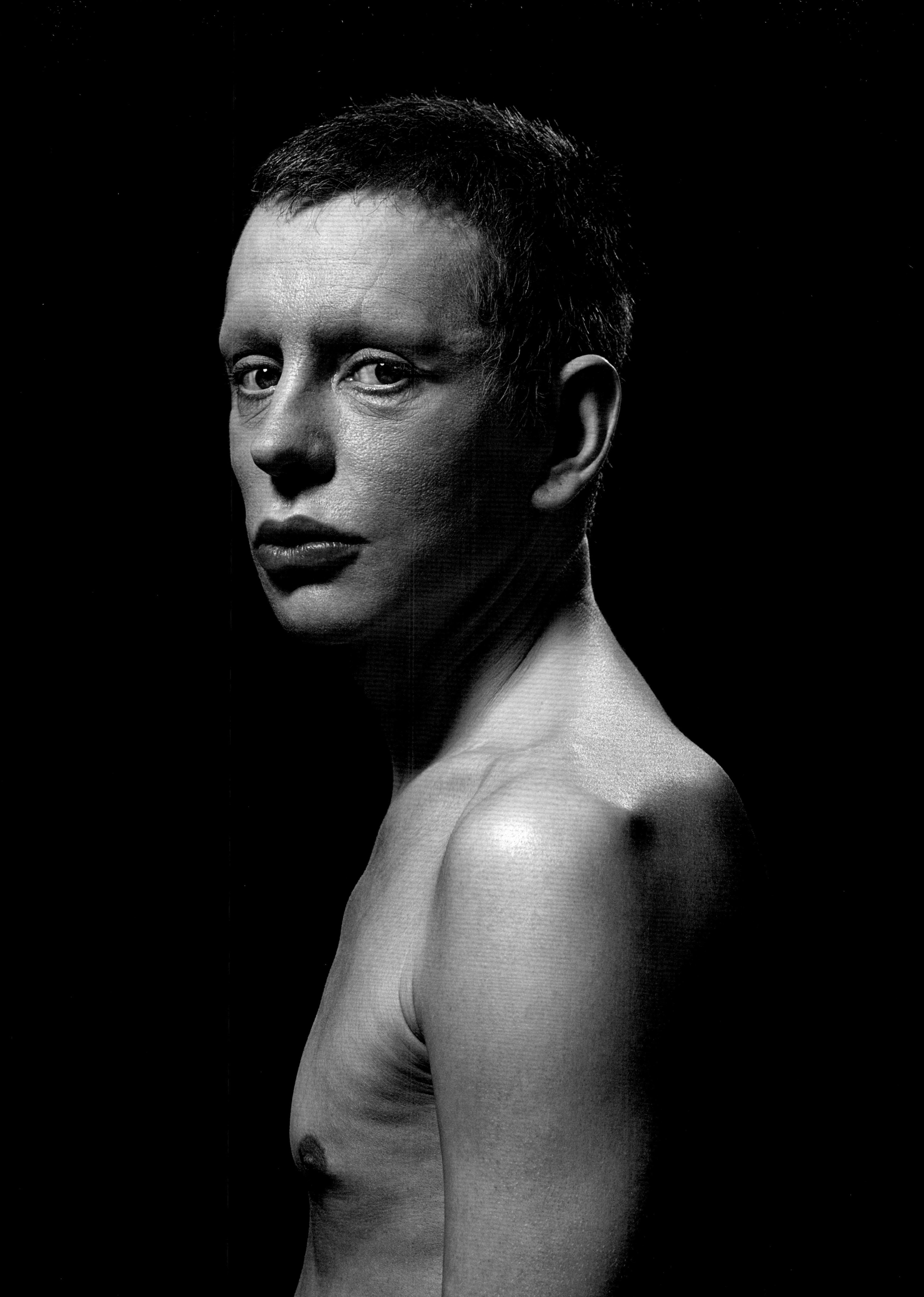

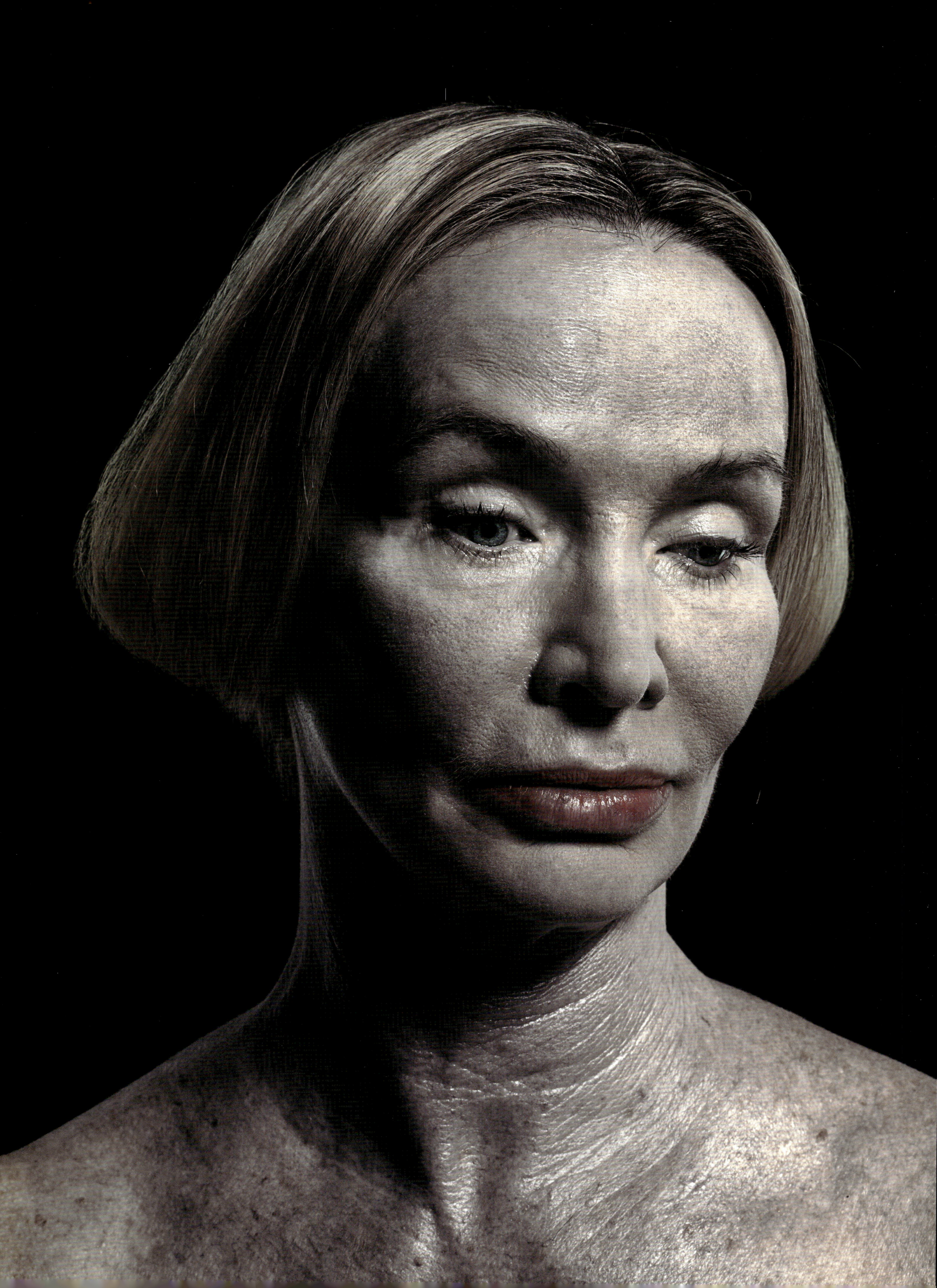

Allanah

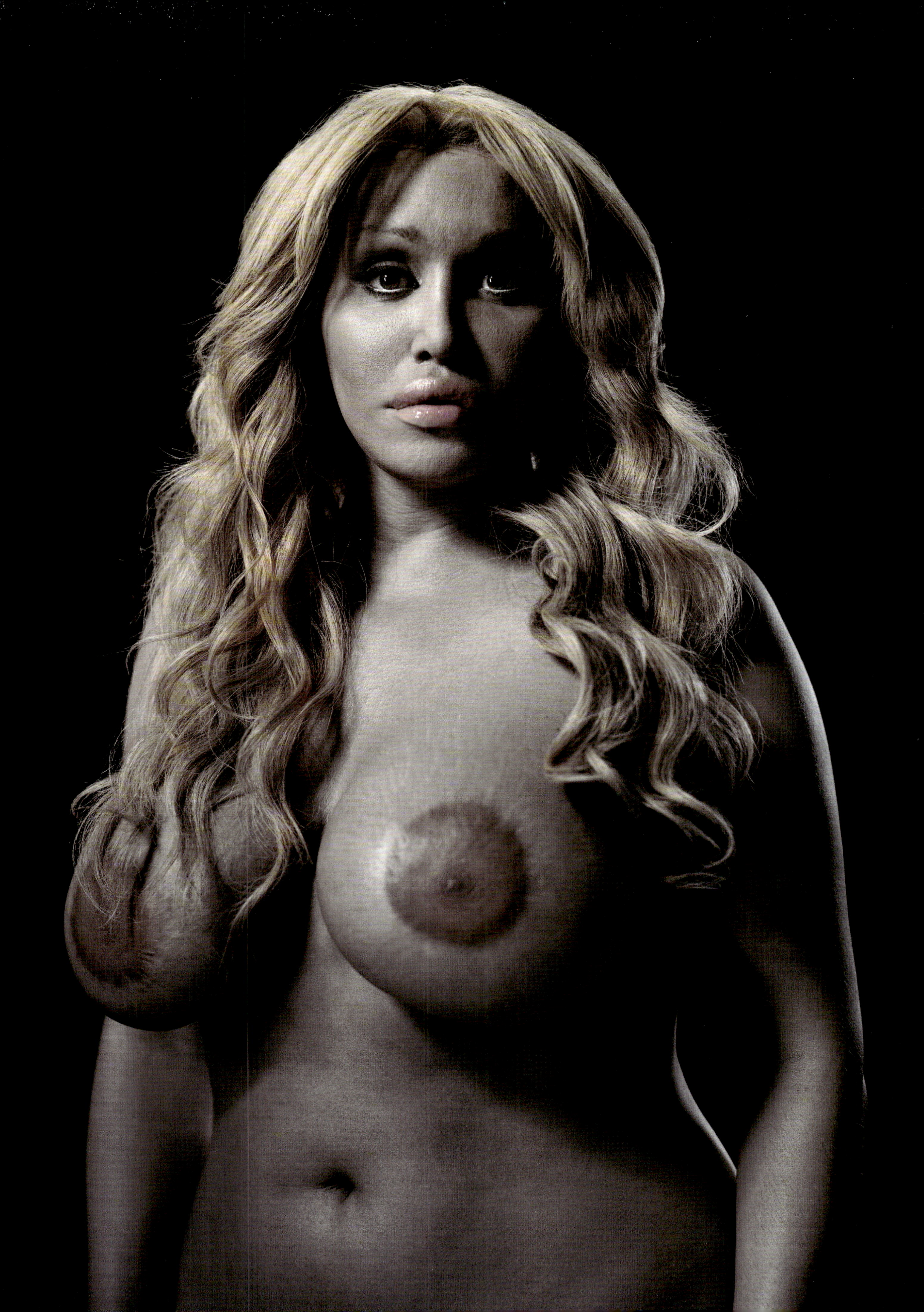

Sonia

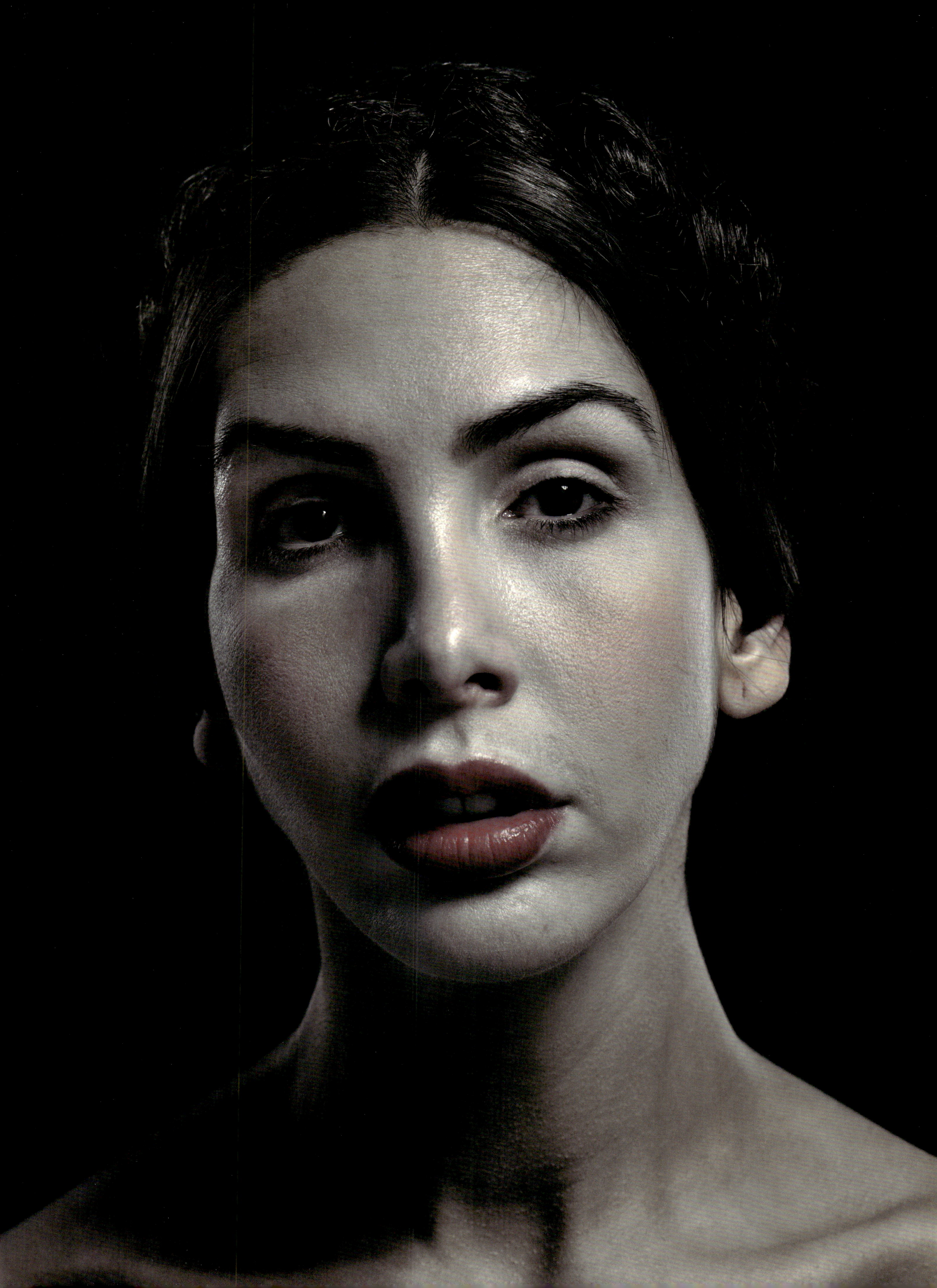

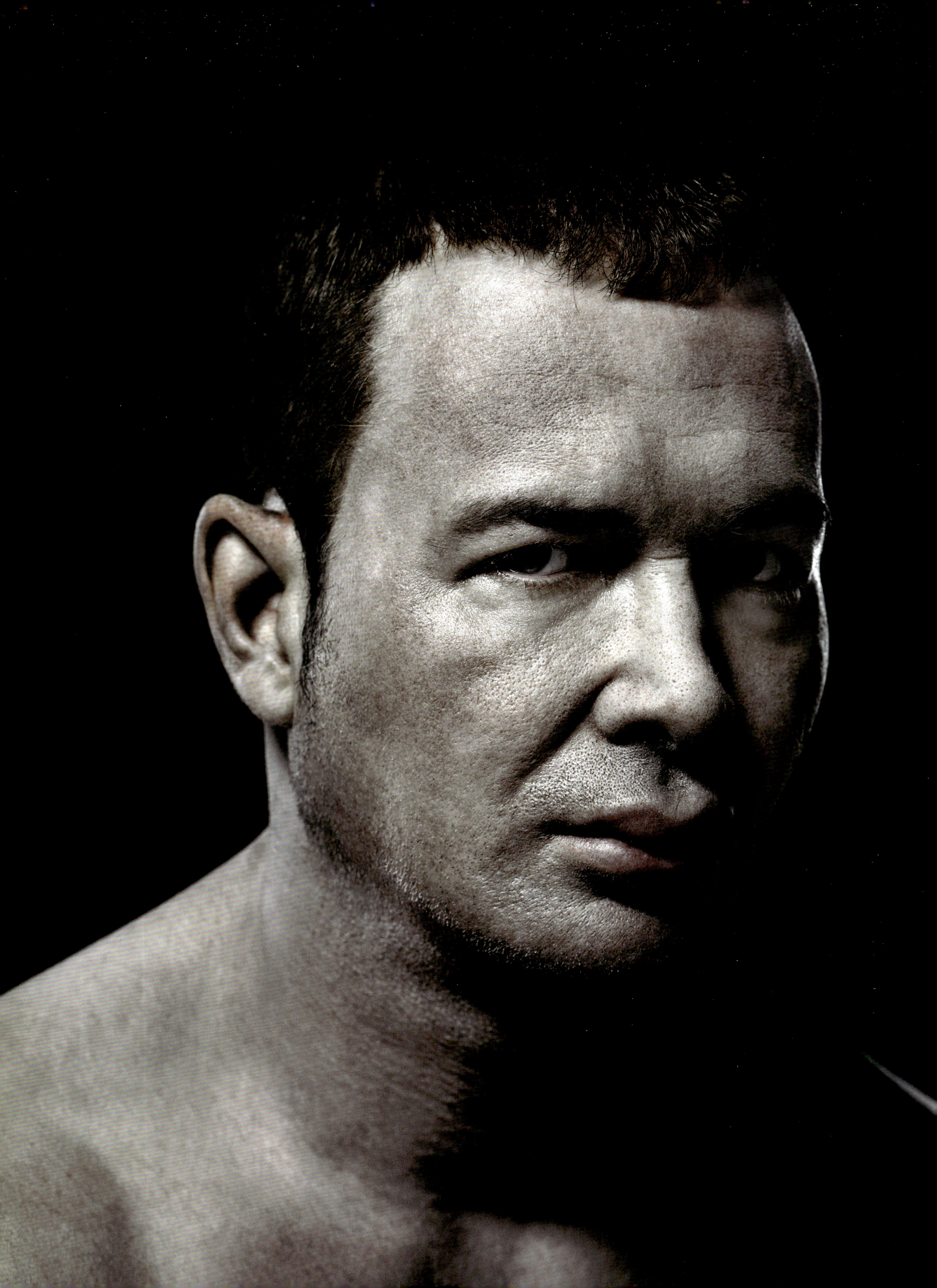

Tyler – *following page* Tiana

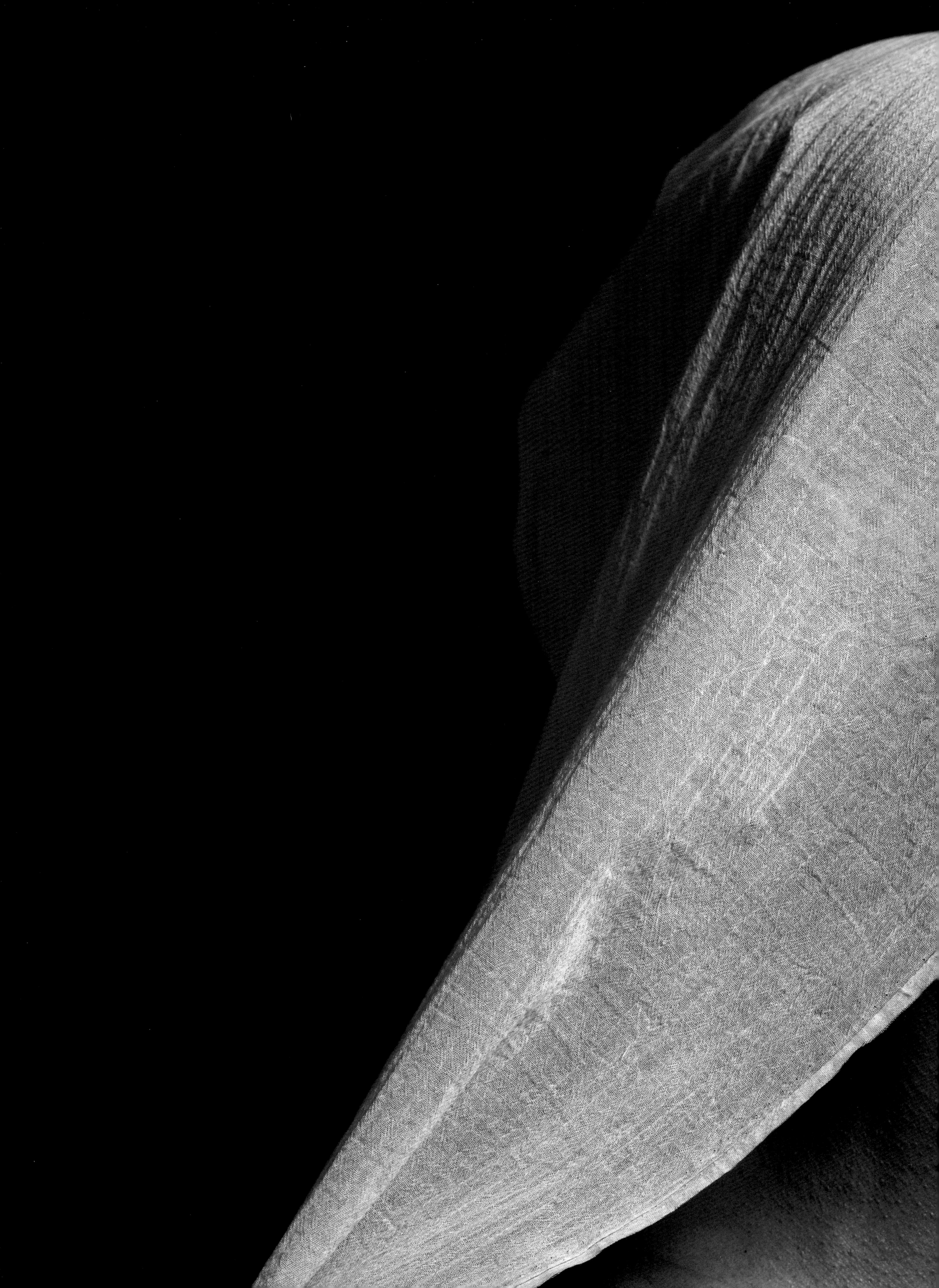

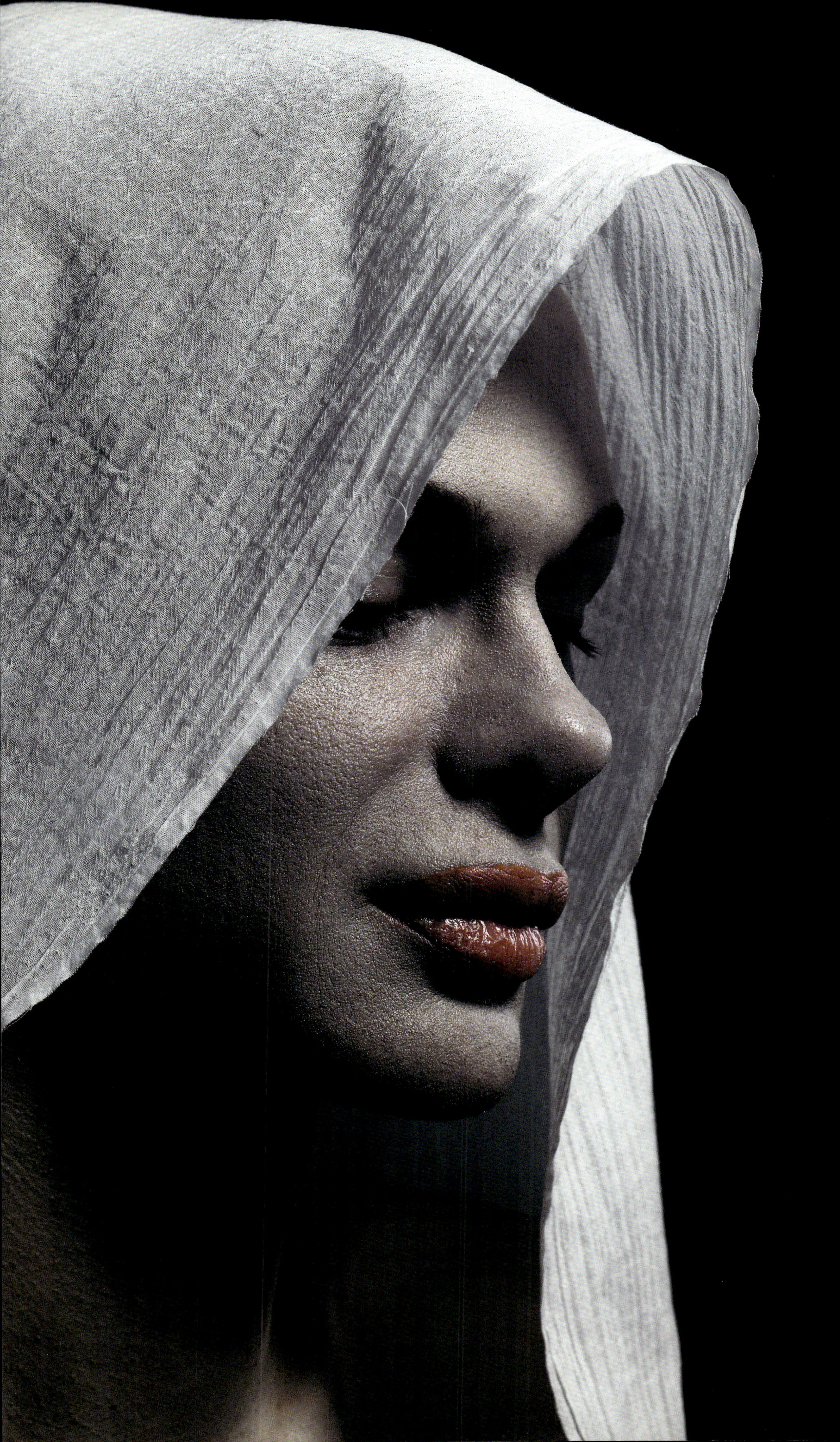

Zander

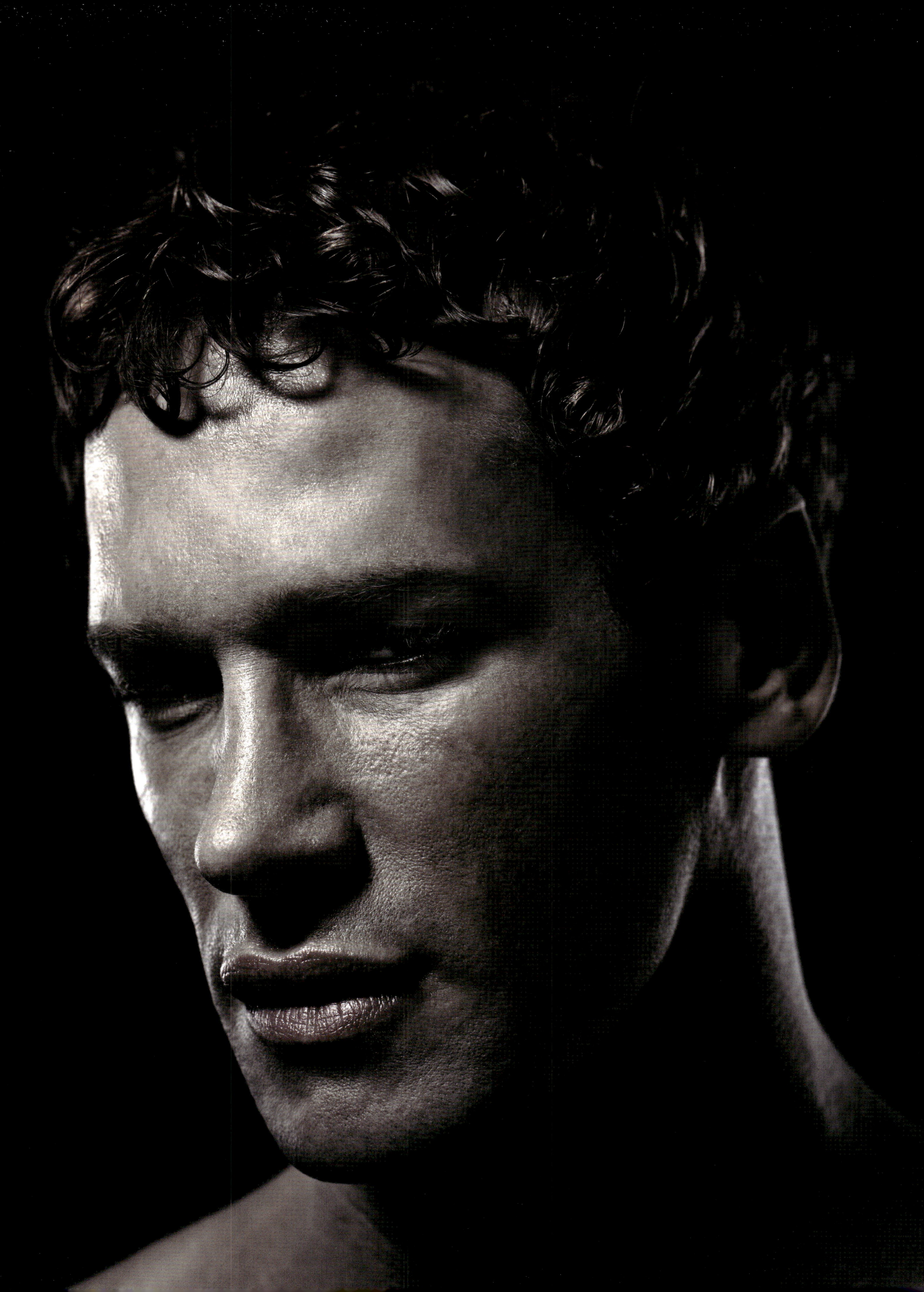

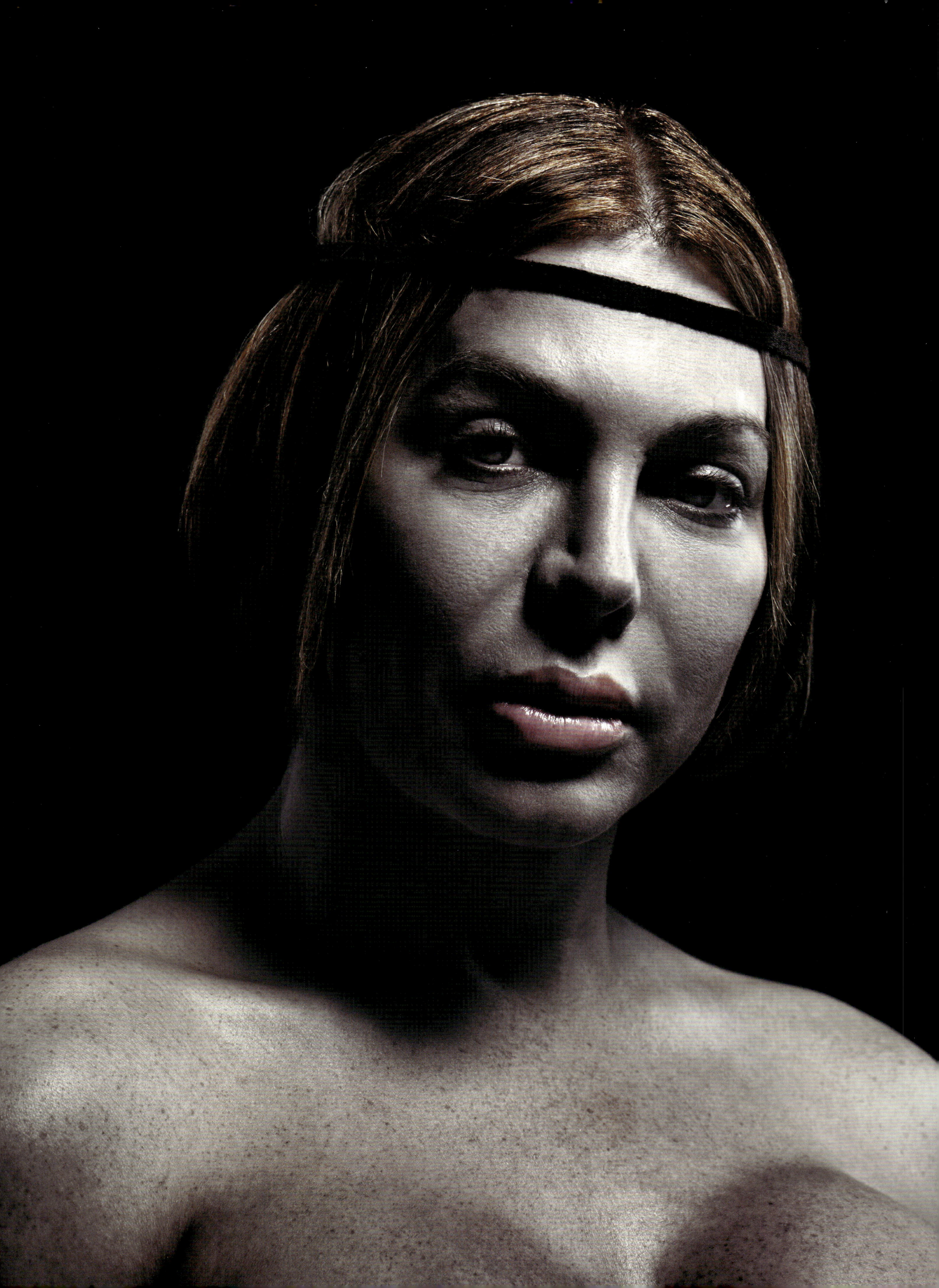

Gina

Steve

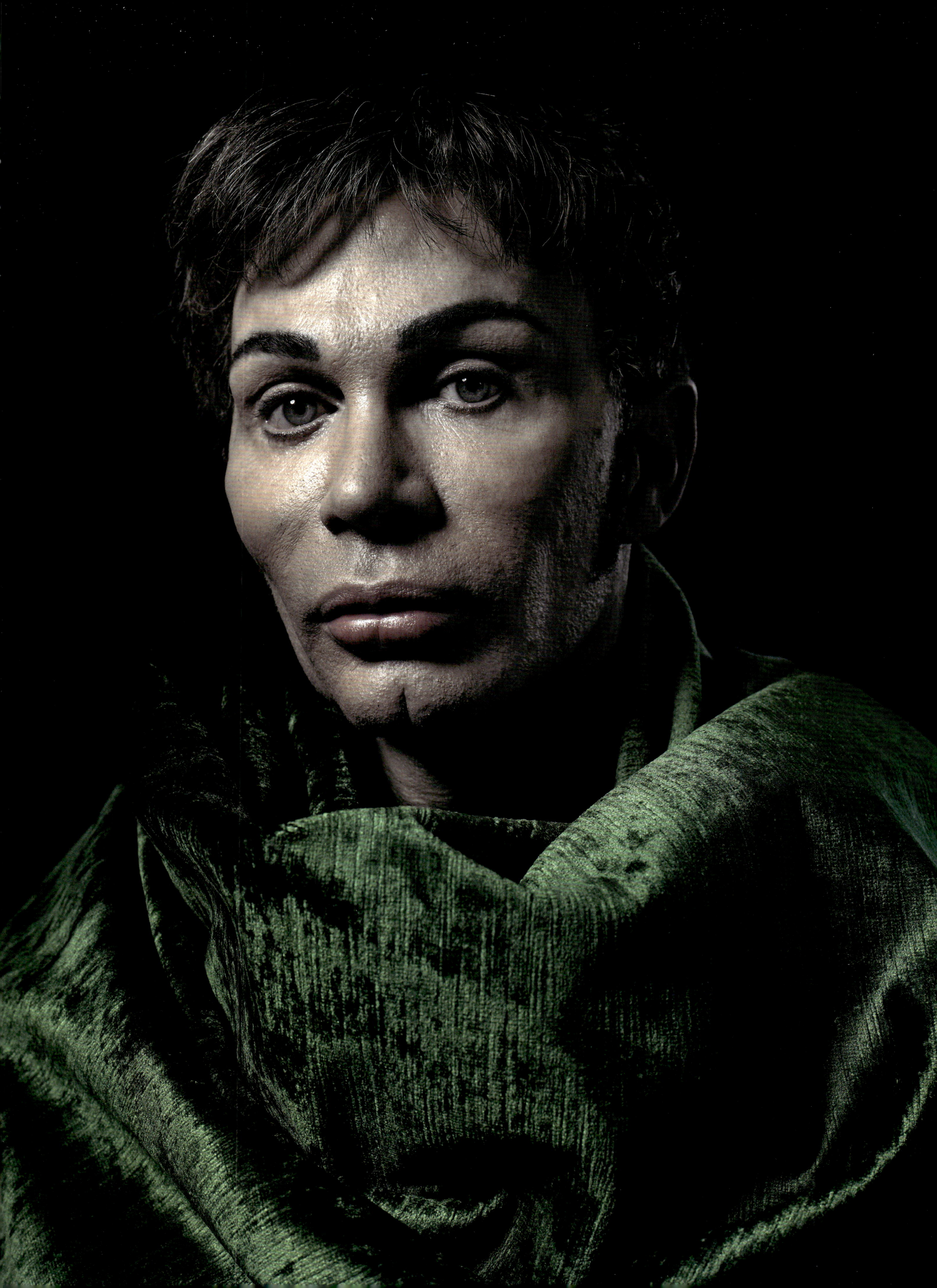

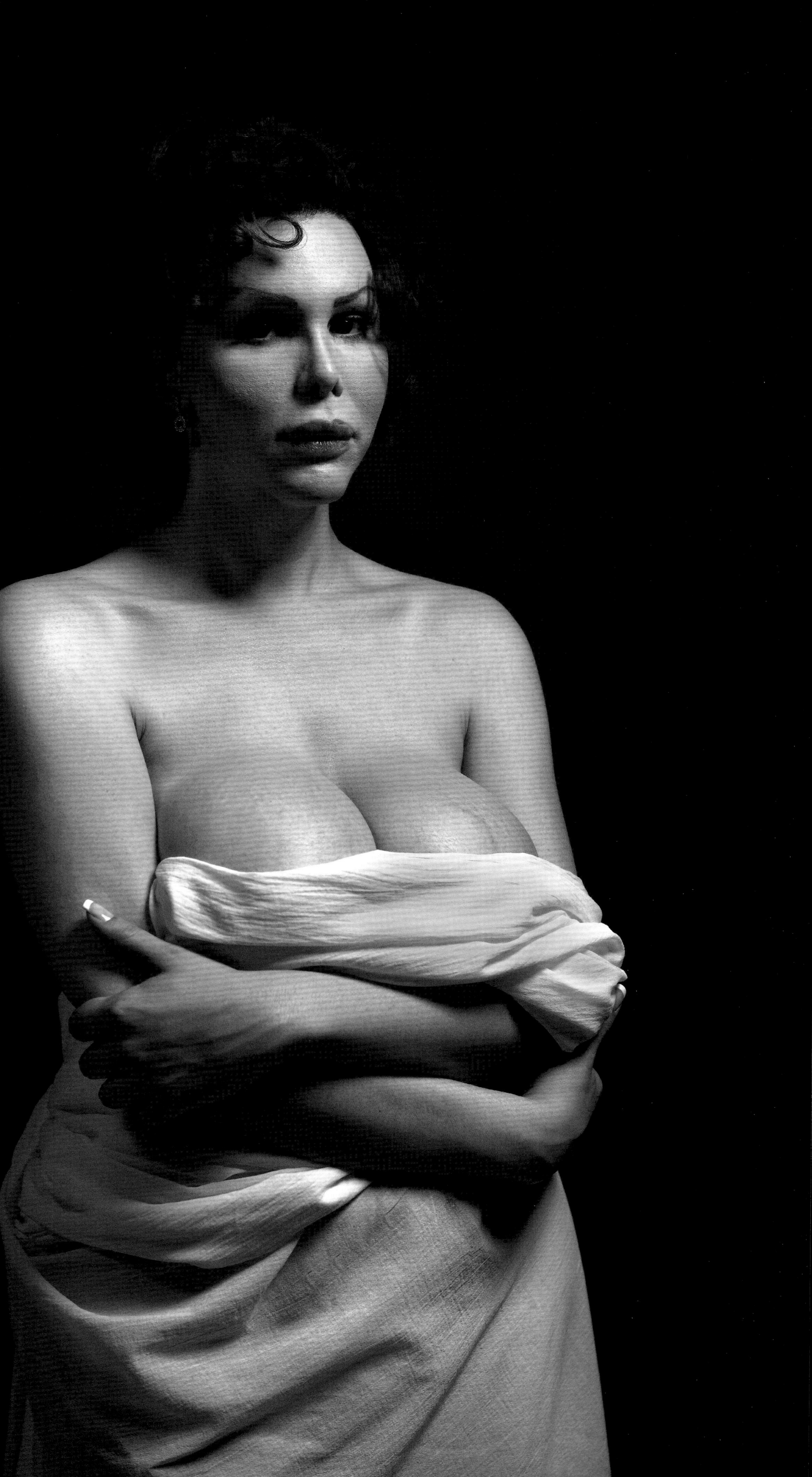

Yvette

A NEW KIND OF BEAUTY

'I am interested in what we define as beauty, when we choose to create ourselves.' – Phillip Toledano

Mister Toledano, as he is known, is a seriously funny fellow, and vice versa. He sees the ironies of life as real and cruel, but he does not despair. He has a chuckle and makes a photograph. Amaze him, amuse him. Life is hard. Here are the pictures. Keep moving.

Having brilliantly addressed aging fathers and sons in *Days with My Father*, here he delivers what he describes as *A New Kind of Beauty*.

The title is exactly right.

'Beauty' is a good looking portfolio of portraits of people who have transformed themselves – recreated themselves. Big time. From soup to ... well, you get it.

These images are remarkably straightforward. The backgrounds are dark, the lighting plays on the skin in a classic chiaroscuro fashion; they have a handsome peachy glow. The sitters, naked or semi-clothed, look out benignly at the viewer.

But the impact of these faces and the bodies is jarring, even, alienating. The sitters' motivations for these enormous changes are undoubtedly personal and deeply felt, but the enormity of that transgressive action challenges us as the viewer to sort out our own ideas about beauty and gender.

The work is neither judgmental nor objective. It is uniquely personal. Toledano is a consummate pro technically and his way of seeing, imaging and imagining is curious without being lurid or sensational. It is respectful.

So what's up?

Beauty gives pleasure to the senses or exalts the spirit. Look it up. A bigger question, is there loveliness here that enthralls, this new kind of beauty?

We can imagine that the ladies: Dina, Yvette, Angel, Allanah, Ava and Gina as well as their opposites, if that is the correct word, Steve, Michael, Jason, and Justin have fulfilled a vision of themselves, perhaps even as they had imagined.

To large extent this 'new kind of beauty' is in the eye of the beheld, not the beholder.

Looking at these works – the photographs and the people – is an uncomfortable exercise for many of us – maybe not all – struck and staggered by the strangeness of this beauty.

These photographs are stunning. We have feelings of real dread encountering these special souls. OH MY GOD! These people may have had their noses and genitals edited. Reassignment, indeed.

All the analogies like feeling buried alive or living underwater don't – excuse me – cut it, as descriptions of the personal histories here. There is the knowable, that these folks have submitted themselves to multiple surgeries, cosmetic adjustments and aggressive hormone treatments, their attempts at bringing order to grave and genuine gender confusion, but beyond that, yikes.

This reaction is not to challenge either the models' or the artist's actions or sympathies but rather to explore the effect this new kind of beauty has on us.

Toledano surrounds his subjects with grace and balance yet does not offer us much of an empathic way in, or out either.

Looking at these images, we have to question how our aesthetic judgments are compromised by our guardedness or discomfort with these seeming distortions, these new proportions. This is different and unfamiliar territory, and that makes us resistant or, after a couple of deep breaths, tentative.

That is what art does sometimes. It is insistent, and it makes us react. It pushes, and we push back.

Mr. T. is artful and cunning. Everything is flesh, refashioned from the shadow. This beauty of reengineering is held in a strange and wonderful light, pinkish yellow, theatrical and severe, bringing the surgically shaped faces and upper bodies into relief. It is distinctly odd.

Breasts, pectorals, designer lips and high cheekbones here are hyperbolic. The choices are self conscious, contemporary, and elective, and that is the new kind of beauty.

Styles change, different body types come into fashion. Body enhancements like tattoos, piercings, scarifications ... bulging biceps and plucked eyebrows describe our tribe. We are conscious of the overwhelming urgency to stay young. It is ironic, as this artist keenly demonstrates that smooth skin and seemingly toned muscles look artificial, and, in fact, unreal and not at all youthful.

This new kind of beauty is a collision of choices.

The most memorable presence and potentially iconic image is Dina with her pillowy lips and important breasts. Such emphatic signifiers of female sexuality are astonishing to behold, full of her outrage and outrageousness.

She, like most of the others, stares us down. The gaze has some diffidence or conventionally pleasant affect. There is no tease, no sense of sensuality. There is also no heat or coolness, no sadness, which might be expected, or happiness either. There is wistfulness, however, an enigmatic but lovely touch. Tiana is particularly poignant, albeit in an old fashioned way.

These portraits will find their own place into the history of Art, into that continuum, with these as the Venuses of Hottentot of today. These are a Cubing of Nature, the ultimate non-traditional Academy studies with some Caravaggio or Velasquez in there too.

This is new, and, yes, kind of beautiful.

W.M. Hunt
July 201

Mr. W.M. Hunt is a champion of photography and his own man.
He thinks Buck Angel is probably important.

with thanks

To Peggy, for introducing me to Dewi, and for
believing in the work the moment she saw it.
To Dewi, of course, same as above.
To my wife, Carla, for putting up with the question
'do you like this one? or this one?' on a daily basis.
To my parents, for giving me the gift of curiosity.
And to everyone in this book – thank you for
allowing me to take your photograph, and for
being so open to this exploration.

First published in the United Kingdom in 2011 by

Dewi Lewis Publishing
8 Broomfield Road, Heaton Moor
Stockport SK4 4ND, England
www.dewilewispublishing.com

All rights reserved

© 2011
for the photographs: Phillip Toledano
for the texts: Phillip Toledano & W.M. Hunt
for this edition: Dewi Lewis Publishing

ISBN: 978-1-907893-10-0

Design and Layout: Dewi Lewis Publishing
Print: EBS, Verona, Italy